Nature's Gentle Cures

Safe & Effective Healing Therapies

Jude C. Williams, MH, ND

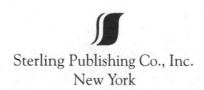

Sterling Publishing Co., Inc.
New York

Edited by Jeanette Green
Herb drawings by Carly Wall

Library of Congress Cataloging-in-Publication Data

Williams, Jude C.
   Nature's gentle cures : safe and effective healing therapies /
Jude C. Williams.
     p.   cm.
   Includes index.
   ISBN 0-8069-9468-1
   1. Herbs—Therapeutic use. 2. Naturopathy. I. Title.
RM666.H33W584   1997
615'.321—dc21   96-49192

1   3   5   7   9   10   8   6   4   2

Published by Sterling Publishing Company, Inc.
387 Park Avenue South, New York, N.Y. 10016
© 1997 by Jude C. Williams
Distributed in Canada by Sterling Publishing
% Canadian Manda Group, One Atlantic Avenue, Suite 105
Toronto, Ontario, Canada M6K 3E7
Distributed in Great Britain and Europe by Cassell PLC
Wellington House, 125 Strand, London WC2R 0BB, England
Distributed in Australia by Capricorn Link (Australia) Pty Ltd.
P.O. Box 6651, Baulkham Hills, Business Centre, NSW 2153, Australia
Manufactured in the United States of America
All rights reserved

Sterling ISBN 0-8069-9468-1

As with any medication, herbal remedies should be taken
under the close supervision of a professional.

For my grandchildren Joshua Todd Williams, Judy C. Williams, and my new great-grandson, David Matthew Williams

Acknowledgments

Thanks to many friends and clients for their help and encouragement. Special thanks to my daughter Carly Wall for her support and her contribution of the botanical drawings. I would also like to give a big thank-you to my editor, Jeanette Green, for help and encouragement through a difficult period.

Contents

Introduction

As microbes mutate and become resistant to yesterday's wonder drugs, many of these drugs today are no longer working as they once did. That's why we need to focus on preventing disease and maintaining the body's immune system with healthful habits and balanced nutrition. Also, many pharmaceutical drugs contain additives and excipients the body does not know how to deal with. Most herbs and natural whole foods, in contrast, contain substances that the body can digest in a natural way.

Modern allopathic medicine often treats just the symptoms and not the root causes of disease. And as people have become more disappointed with pharmaceutical drug cures, they have returned to time-honored herbal remedies. Herbs work slowly but effectively in helping the body defend itself against disease. Herbs naturally offer a more complex resource than single-chemical drugs or pill-form extracts. In them are found not only vital nutrients but thousands of phytochemicals (*phyto-* means "plant") that defend the body against carcinogens and other disease-causing substances. Over 10,000 are in the tomato alone.

Biologically active substances, the phytochemicals in plants give them color, flavor, and natural disease resistance. They include flavonoids, genistein, indoles, saponins, P-coumaric acid, phenethyl isothiocyanate, and many more chemicals that contribute to both the prevention and cure of disease. Medicinal herbs as well as common fruits, vegetables, grains, and legumes contain these phytochemicals in abundance. Berries, apricots, grapes, onions, kale, cabbage, tomatoes, and garlic block tumor growth and neutralize carcinogens, due not simply to the vital nutrients they supply but to their phytochemicals.

We know that nutrients work synergistically and that a deficiency of one can affect the absorption and assimilation of other vitamins and minerals. The many phytochemicals in herbs appear to work that way, too. That's why pharmaceutical drugs drawn from a single source found within an herb seem to fail to offer the body the full spectrum of benefits gained from ingesting the herb itself. Recognized medicinal herbs, like many plants, have built-in checks and balances of phytochemicals that allow them to flourish.

We have much to learn. Recent studies have found that bitter substances in some fruits protect them against invaders like fruit-eating fungi. This may help explain why some sweet-tasting hybrid fruits we favor spoil more quickly than other fruits found in the wild. It may also explain why these fruits do not protect us as well from invading microbes and disease.

At one time, foods we ate and herbs used for natural healing contained all the nutrients necessary for good health. But soils worldwide have been depleted of vital nutrients, and we now reap that devalued harvest planted decades ago. We compound the problem with widespread use of pesticides and other chemicals used to control our crops and quicken the growth of livestock. Environmental pollutants and toxins also overwork the body's immune system. We need to return to a healthful diet and to nourish body, mind, and spirit to maintain optimal health. A healthy body naturally responds quickly to any disorder.

It takes many years of abuse and improper nutrition for a serious illness, like colon cancer, to develop. Just think about it. The body fights chronic nutritional deficiencies for as long as twenty years before it becomes so weakened that cancer cells thrive.

We are responsible for our own health. A wholesome, complete diet balanced with exercise and rest is just the first step toward having a healthy body, mind, and spirit.

Herbal Medicine

In order to survive, ancient peoples needed to learn the secrets of nature. They achieved much of this by observation and experimentation. They watched as wild and domesticated animals chose certain plants for their daily diet and turned to others when ill. And they hoped to discover methods for reading plants—the book of nature—to understand their possible uses to treat human diseases.

In the 16th century, Swiss alchemist and physician Paracelsus codified a doctrine of signatures that could help herbalists understand the functions of different herbs by observing their signature, or appearance. Many herbalists today still rely on this ancient identification system to discover both traditional and vital new uses of given herbs. I personally ascribe to this system.

Plants with blue flowers, like passionflower, lavender, valerian, and sage, are used as sedatives. Yellow flowers indicate herbs useful for cleaning the urinary tract. White flowers advise us that the herb will serve as a tonic for the whole body. And red flowers advertise the plant's use as a blood cleanser. This telltale color may also appear on the plant's leaves, root, or stem. The burdock stem, for instance, is red, and it has long been used as a blood purifier and for cancer remedies. Silverweed's root produces a reddish dye and the plant resembles a dried strawberry. It is helpful for bleeding gums, bleeding piles, and as an astringent. It also helps stop internal bleeding.

The names, like *skullcap, pleurisy root, cancer root,* and *feverfew,* given to herbs by our forebears also indicate their probable use.

The plant's growing conditions are observed for intuiting the herb's possible powers. Plants that thrive in gravel, like mullein, might be helpful in removing stones from the gallbladder or kidneys. They are also thought helpful in cleaning the bronchial and alimentary systems.

Herbs that thrive in swampy areas are considered to be helpful for asthma, coughs, and colds. Willow and boneset, for instance, are thought to reduce mucus buildup.

Prickly herbs and herbs with sharp thorns, like hawthorn, are used to treat sharp pain and conditions like angina. Soft-textured herbs help treat swollen, inflamed parts of the body and may be helpful for the chest or for colds.

But all herbs do not bear a signature. And we must divine through experimentation and study what they can do. We continue to discover new herbs found in vanishing rain forests and other parts of the globe. And these herbs may one day become vital to our survival, just as herbs were for our distant forebears.

When using this book as a health guide, please keep in mind that each of us has a different tolerance to certain substances. Biochemists refer to this as biochemical individuality. What may work for me may not work for you. Begin trying small amounts of the recommended herb(s) before taking larger doses to treat an ailment. If you have an allergic reaction, stop taking the herb immediately. Many other herbs may serve the same purpose.

Also, many people think if a little helps, then a lot would do the trick better and faster. But this is not true. Most herbal remedies are intended for short-term use. Too much of a good thing, like echinacea or penicillin, will stop working. And too much could also make you ill, just as eating a whole pie could. Remember: HERBS MUST BE USED WITH CAUTION. Just as you should not take a prescription medication heedlessly, you must not take herbal remedies heedlessly. Read all instructions related to the particular herb and heed all cautions.

Herbs take time to work, so continue any suggested remedy for at least three months unless stated otherwise. We must understand that herbs cannot be miracle cures. Herbs by themselves do not heal, just as drugs do not heal, and physicians cannot heal. By ingesting an herb, you are fueling your body with necessary nutrients and phytochemicals so that it can heal itself.

Consult your physician before beginning any of the herbal remedies described in this book. Many physicians are willing to work with you when you use natural remedies. Also, it's unwise to stop taking current medications. Have your physician monitor your progress before attempting to change any medications. You may even be able to convert your physician to using more natural means to treat illnesses because of your steady improvement.

How to Prepare Herbs

Some herbs may be used directly as tea leaves. Others work best in tinctures that steep for weeks. And still others work best when powdered. See the recipe that appears most useful for your ailment and follow directions. Also, review all herbs contained in the recipe (check index) to make sure that they are not contraindicated for your particular illness.

Many herbs presented in these chapters can be used alone or combined with other herbs in teas, tinctures, infusions, poultices, and more. A given herb may be helpful for more than one ailment. But some herbs, like licorice root or Siberian ginseng, must be avoided if you have high blood pressure, for instance. So, you would not want to take it to treat another disorder if your blood pressure is a problem. That's why it's important to read all cautions associated with any herb.

Some herbs are intended for short-term use only, others for acute crisis, and still others may be safe to take for an extended time. Again, read all directions carefully and consult a qualified physician to monitor your progress on any herbal regimen.

Herbal Teas Use about 1 to 3 teaspoons of herb(s) per cup of boiling water. Allow the herb to steep in a cup or pot for at least 5 minutes, but no longer than 10 minutes. If you prefer a stronger tea, use more of the herb(s). Many teas may be used daily as tonics. This method is practical for herbs that may be too strong to take in other forms. Add honey to sweeten, if you wish. Never gulp medicinal teas; take them in slow, warm sips.

Tinctures Use 1 to 3 ounces of herb with 1 pint to 1 quart of brandy or vodka. Allow the herb mixture to steep for two to several weeks. Tinctures keep for a long period of time. They can be added to 1 cup of boiling water for a tea. The alcohol evaporates when boiling water is added. For serious illness, the tincture may be taken directly under the tongue for quick absorption by the body.

Infusions Infusions use the leaves, flowers, or other delicate parts of the plant. The plant is steeped, not boiled, for about 5 minutes in hot water. This will prevent the herb's benefits from being destroyed by the heat.

Powders Use a mortar and pestle to grind the herb, or simply buy a small coffee grinder and use it exclusively for the purpose. Powders may be used in teas, tinctures, capsules, poultices, or wherever called for.

Syrups Honey or glycerin added to the herb forms a sugar that can be boiled. This increases the shelf life of the herb and makes it easy to take, especially if the herb is bitter. A syrup may be added to boiling water for a tea or taken directly by the teaspoon.

Salves You can make a salve with the herb by adding vegetable oil to it. Use beeswax to achieve the consistency you want.

Compresses and Poultices Mix the powdered herb with a little water to form a paste and apply the paste to loosely woven clean cloth, like cotton or muslin. Apply the poultice to the skin of the affected area after cleansing it with soap and water, then with hydrogen peroxide. Place a cloth over the poultice to retain heat. You can use a cloth soaked in the heated liquid herbal paste. Change the poultice often. Thoroughly wash the area when the poultice is finally removed.

Herb Vinegars　Herbs can be preserved and used in an apple cider vinegar. Allow the mixture (1 to 3 ounces of herb with 1 pint to 1 quart of vinegar) to stand two or more weeks.

Decoctions　These teas, made from the herb's bark, root, seeds, or berries, are not boiled. They are simmered for long periods of time to extract the herb's benefits.

Special Cautions

Do not give herbs to young children, and it's best to avoid herbs during pregnancy. Pregnant women must be especially careful to avoid **barberry, black cohosh, blue cohosh, boneset, cat's claw, celery, cinnamon, comfrey, feverfew, goldenseal, licorice, passionflower, pennyroyal, rhubarb,** and **wormwood.**

Although relatively safe, the herbs **damiana, bilberry (blueberry), burdock, peppermint, sage, St.-John's-wort,** and **willow** may interfere with the body's absorption of iron and other minerals.

Herbs in this book have a long history of beneficial use in herbal medicine. But you must exercise extra caution in the use of **chaparral, comfrey, elder, ephedra, hydrangea, licorice, lobelia, Siberian ginseng,** and **wild cherry.** Some may have extremely dangerous side effects: depressed blood pressure, difficulty breathing, gastrointestinal disturbances, liver damage, kidney disorders, rapid heartbeat, stroke, memory loss, psychosis, paralysis, coma, and even death. **Chaparral** and **comfrey** are usually recommended for external use only. Parts of **elder, hydrangea,** and **wild cherry** plants are toxic. Use all these herbs only for the condition indicated and only under close medical supervision.

No herb should be taken casually. Consult a physician before beginning any herbal regimen and review all contraindications. Do not exceed the recommended dose or treatment period. Do not use the herb(s) if you have an allergic or other adverse reaction. If you experience skin rash, hives, itching, redness, dizziness, fever, disorientation or agitation, digestive upset, abdominal cramps, swelling, or any unusual reaction, discontinue the herb(s) immediately. Flush the whole system with apple juice.

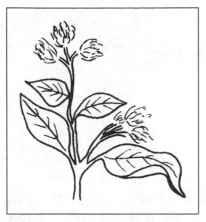

Burdock

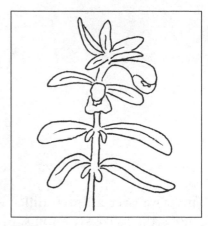

Skullcap

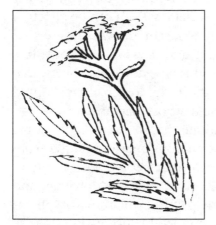

Valerian

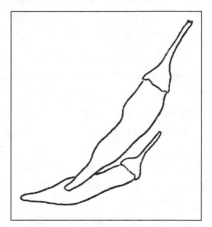

Cayenne Pepper

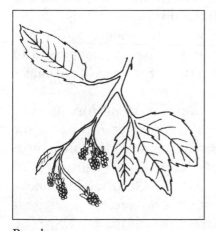

Raspberry

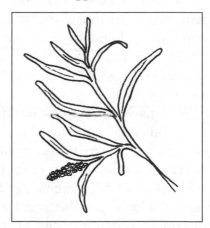

Willow

1. Arthritis

There are over a dozen different types of arthritis and diseases that cause arthritislike symptoms. Many affect the movement of the joints and cartilage, and some affect the bone. Arthritis can take many different forms. Any part of the body's skeletal system can be affected. The most common form of arthritis is **osteoarthritis,** which is related to the wear and tear of joints due to aging and stress on the body. It is considered a degenerative joint disease. This type normally affects people over age 40; only rarely does it affect children. In the United States, an estimated 15.8 million people have osteoarthritis.

Rheumatoid arthritis, an autoimmune disease, can affect people of all ages, including children. Over 2.2 million Americans suffer from rheumatoid arthritis. Research has shown that people with rheumatoid arthritis have lower than average levels of folic acid, protein, and zinc. This form of arthritis is particularly painful. Inflammatory in nature, it involves the synovial joints, surrounded by lubricating fluid.

Systemic lupus erythematosus, a malfunction of the immune system, mimics rheumatoid arthritis. With this disease, the joints may become painful and swollen, but it is not the crippling disorder that rheumatoid arthritis is. Women with lupus outnumber men eight to one. About 200,000 people are afflicted with it in the United States alone.

Arthritis is linked to the health of the blood and circulatory systems; so, good circulation has a lot to do with treatment of arthritis. If the condition is severe, bedrest is important during periods of inflammation to avoid further damage to the joints. Ice packs over a towel for 20 minutes help relieve swelling and reduce damage. Get up and resume as normal a life as possible when inflammation is not present. Exercise is important in both prevention and treatment of arthritis and helps you to improve muscle strength and the joints' fluidity of motion.

Joint problems are nearly always accompanied by intestinal or stomach distress. Dry stools, gas, and bloating are common. When too much acid is present in the body, this is usually caused by lack of sodium. Sodium can be burned out by acids. Because we store sodium in the stomach wall, this can cause difficulties in assimilation and elimination if it is depleted. When sodium absorption is poor we do not have a proper balance of electrolytes in the gastrointestinal system. Sodium is found as a carbonate in the blood, where it is essential to contributing to the blood's alkalinity. When you have a backache caused by lifting or strain and your back "goes out," this is caused by lack of sodium in the diet.

Chlorine has been found in every tissue in the body, but it is mainly in the blood as sodium chloride. Chlorine occurs in combination with sodium, potassium, and calcium.

Some believe we do not need calcium in the diet because it settles in the joints. We erroneously conclude that we have too much calcium in the body. In fact, calcium that settles in the joints is caused by the lack of sodium and other minerals in the area. The lack of sodium in the body actually causes this deposit of calcium in the joints. Lack of calcium in turn causes the bones to break down. Thus, those who suffer from arthritis need much more sodium in their diet than the average person in order to assimilate the calcium needed to fortify the bones. Sodium is the chemical material needed to soften any hard material that may settle in the joints.

Gout is believed to be caused by a long habit of alcohol consumption and meat or a high-protein intake. Alcohol can disturb normal kidney function, preventing the kidneys from processing uric acid. The uric acid then enters the bloodstream and settles in the joints. That's why protein and alcohol intake must be cut when treating gout.

Vitamin C in large amounts seems to stimulate recuperation from arthritis and gout, so it would be helpful to include large amounts of citrus fruits, especially oranges and limes, in your daily diet. Most people suffering from gout seem to suffer from a vitamin C deficiency.

Sodium has to be restored to the affected joints. Diet plays an important part in treatment of any form of arthritis, but it is most important in the treatment of gout. Exercise, proper diet, fresh air, and sunshine also play a central role in treatment. Suffering from overwork, lacking hobbies different from your vocation, experiencing stress, being divorced from nature, and not having enough play lead to many physical disorders and diseases, including all forms of arthritis.

Whether we deal with arthritis, gout, lupus erythematosis, osteoarthritis, or rheumatoid arthritis, we are dealing with the same problem. All these diseases are brought about by a nutritional shortage in the body.

For foods and herbs high in sodium, calcium, and potassium, check the lists in chapter 10. These foods are essential to your daily diet.

RECOMMENDED NUTRIENTS

For arthritis, gout, and lupus erythematosus, include these nutrients in your diet: sodium, chlorine, calcium, potassium, and vitamin C. If you have gout, avoid alcohol and excess protein in the diet. For arthritis, avoid nightshade vegetables (tomatoes, peppers, eggplant, white potato), do not take an iron supplement, and avoid extra vitamin D in milk. Consult foods high in the recommended nutrients for arthritislike conditions in chapter 10. Investigate any possible food allergies.

HELPFUL HERBS

Herbs that may be helpful in the treatment of arthritis, systemic lupus erythematosus, and gout include: apple pectin, burdock, sassafras, violet, valerian, ginger, cayenne pepper, alfalfa seeds, chaparral, licorice root, willow, celery seed, slippery elm, skullcap, raspberry, butcher's broom, black cohosh, and Joe-pye weed.

APPLE PECTIN
Pyrus malus

SIGNATURE: The red color of the fruit is apple's signature.

Apples contain malic and tartaric acids, and this denotes use as a treatment for neutralizing waste products. Crab apples are particularly high in pectin.

Apple pectin helps protect the body from disease by flushing out toxins. Pectin binds with bile acids and helps decrease fat absorption.

Most fruit sugars are treated as predigested food and reach the bloodstream quickly. The fruit acid helps neutralize waste products of rheumatism, gout, and arthritis. Never peel an apple, because the nutrients of the fruit are just beneath and in the peel.

It is helpful to flush the gastrointestinal system before using remedies to treat arthritis. Apple pectin helps cleanse and flush the digestive system and prepares the body to assimilate and use needed herbs and vegetables.

APPLE CIDER POULTICE

Apple cider is also a great poultice for swollen joints. Mix together 2 quarts of apple cider vinegar, 4 ounces of mullein, $\frac{1}{4}$ ounce of cayenne pepper, and $\frac{1}{2}$ ounce of lobelia. Reduce heat after mixture reaches a boil and simmer for 30 minutes. Strain and soak a clean cloth in the resulting liquid. Place it over the affected joint and keep warm. Replace with a hot poultice as needed.

VALERIAN
Valeriana officinalis

OTHER NAMES: Setwall, phu, Jacob's ladder, garden heliotrope, Greek valerian, great valerian, American valerian, lady's slippers, garden valerian, water valerian, capon's tail, English valerian, all heal, German valerian, and amantella.
PART USED: Root.
SIGNATURE: The fine roots growing from the short root stalks are said to be similar to the human brain structure.

Valerian has an influence on the cerebrospinal system, so it is helpful for treatment of arthritis since it allows the body to relax. The herb contains magnesium, camphene, formic acid, valeric acid, and valerine. It acts as a sedative, relieves muscle spasms, and improves circulation.

This herb should be used with other herbs. Some people are very sensitive to the effects of valerian and go to sleep immediately. If you take the herb during working hours, this can create a problem. Here's a good mixture for a valerian capsule.

VALERIAN CAPSULES

1 tablespoon of powdered valerian
1 tablespoon of powdered licorice root
1 tablespoon of powdered butcher's broom
1 tablespoon of powdered cayenne or ginger

Mix the powdered herbs and fill #00 capsules. Take 2 capsules three times daily.

VALERIAN TEA

Make a tea by adding 1 ounce of valerian root to 1 pint of boiling water. Simmer for ten minutes, covered. Strain and add 2 ounces of honey or glycerin to preserve the fluid. Drink several times daily and before bedtime.

ALFALFA
Medicago sativa

PART USED: Flowers, leaves, petals, and sprouts.

Alfalfa contains saponin, which suggests it has some steroid properties. It is also useful for cellular detoxification due to its fiber content. The herb alkalizes and detoxifies the body. It is good for anemia, bone and joint disorders, skin disorders, and colon and digestive disorders.

Alfalfa has high nutritional value, and for this reason alone it can be used as a treatment. It contains essential amino acids, calcium, copper, iron, magnesium, phosphorus, potassium, sodium, sulfur, and zinc. It also contains beta-carotene, and vitamins A, C, D, E, and K as well as B complex.

CELERY SEED
Apium Graveolens

PART USED: The seeds, leaves, and stems.
SIGNATURE: The signature of the plant includes stems that are thick and juicy, a pale green color, and thick seeds. When the base is cut, it appears diaphragmlike.

Celery has been used for centuries as a diuretic and blood cleanser, so it is good for use as a treatment for arthritis, gout, and rheumatism. Studies have shown that celery seed has some insulinlike activity. Celery seed contains iron, as well as vitamins A, B complex, and C. It is an antioxidant and acts as a sedative. It's good for arthritis because it relieves muscle cramps. Celery is also good for kidney disorders. Do not use during pregnancy.

CELERY SEED TEA

Make an infusion by pouring 1 pint of boiling water over $1/2$ ounce of celery seed. Cover and let steep until cool. Strain and bottle. Store in the refrigerator. Take 1 to 3 tablespoons three times daily.

CHAPARRAL
Larrea divaricata

OTHER NAMES: Chaparro, greasewood, dwarf evergreen oak, creosote bush.
PART USED: The stem and leaves.

Chaparral contains a small amount of sterols. It also contains protein, sucrose, gums, resins, sulfur, sodium, and zinc. It acts as a free-radical scavenger and purifies the blood. This bitter herb has been used to treat everything from cancer, skin conditions, arthritis, prostate and kidney disorders, to throat and bronchial conditions. It protects against sun exposure and radiation.

According to scientific studies and Native American medicine, chaparral contains antirheumatoid properties. Nordihydroquaiaretic acid (NDGA) has analgesic (pain reliever) and vasodepressant (circulation-depressing) properties. NDGA, the primary constituent of chaparral, also increases ascorbic acid levels in the adrenal glands. NDGA stimulates the process by which cells utilize foods for energy.

Caution: Taking chaparral in large doses or for long periods can cause liver damage. It is considered safe for external use.

CHAPARRAL TEA

To prepare a tea, place 2 tablespoons of chaparral in a quart jar. Pour 1 quart of boiling water over the herb and let stand overnight. Do not strain, refrigerate, or remove the surface settlement. Drink 1 cup before each meal and before bedtime.

LICORICE ROOT
Glycyrrhiza glabra

OTHER NAMES: Sweetwood, cascarilla.
PART USED: The root.
SIGNATURE: The sweet taste, slightly mucilaginous texture, and the long root are signatures of this plant.

Licorice root is used to treat arthritis because it contains substantial antiarthritic properties. The anti-inflammatory effect occurs because the herb nourishes the adrenal glands, which then release corticosteroids. Licorice root is as effective as hydrocortisone, without the side effects. Studies have shown that licorice stimulates the production of interferon. It is beneficial to the digestive tract and to allergic disorders and asthma. It soothes bronchitis.

The herb contains biotin, choline, folic acid, inositol, lecithin, manganese, pantothenic acid, PABA, phosphorus, protein, and vitamins B_1, B_2, B_3, B_6, and E.

You can add licorice root to capsules, tinctures, or teas as an aid in treating arthritis.

Caution: If you have high blood pressure, do not use this herb.

CAYENNE PEPPER
Capsicum annuum

OTHER NAMES: Capsicum, hot pepper, chili pepper, long pepper, red pepper.
PART USED: The fruit.
SIGNATURE: The red color of the pepper is its signature.

Cayenne pepper has long been used as a blood purifier. It also destroys bacteria that are in the blood. It acts as a diaphoretic that stimulates the excretion of waste from the body through perspiration. Cayenne improves circulation and acts as a catalyst, assuring a fast delivery of other important properties from other herbs. It is used as a treatment for arthritis, pleurisy, and nausea.

Cayenne contains vitamin C, minerals, and alphatocopherols, nutrients important for the health of the circulatory system. It also contains aspaicine, capsaicin, capsanthine, capsico, PABA, and vitamins B_1, B_2, B_3, B_5, B_6, and B_9.

CAYENNE PEPPER TEA

Add $^1/_2$ teaspoon of cayenne pepper to 1 cup warm water for a tea. Stir and drink as quickly as possible.

Caution: Although it has been used to treat arthritis since it stimulates circulation and acts as a catalyst for other herbs, cayenne pepper, like other nightshade family plants, contains solanine, which creates an enzyme that irritates joints. About 10 percent of the population is allergic to the solanine in nightshade-family (Solanaceae) vegetables (white potatoes, tomatoes, peppers, eggplant, zucchini, and more). Tobacco is also a member of this family. This allergy has been linked with arthritislike symptoms.

JOE-PYE WEED
Eupatorium purpureum

OTHER NAMES: Gravel root, swamp root, purple boneset, boneset, trumpet weed, queen-of-the-meadow.
PART USED: The whole plant can be used, but the roots are most often used for medicinal remedies. The flowers are used for diuretic and tonic purposes.
SIGNATURE: The plant grows in wet, swampy, or rich soil.

Joe-Pye weed is often used as a substitute for white boneset (*Eupatorium perfoliatum*). It is often mistaken for the boneset herb. But you can tell the difference from the bloom and leaves of the plants. Boneset has a white bloom, and the leaves are joined at the plant's stem. Joe-Pye weed has a purple bloom and grows much taller than boneset.

The root, made into a strong decoction, is used in any condition where there are uric-acid deposits. It is useful in treatment of joint stiffness, gout, and rheumatism. It contains euparin and eupurpurin.

To prepare an infusion of Joe-Pye weed, place 2 ounces of the root in 2 pints of water. Allow it to stand for several hours before bringing to a boil and quickly reducing to a simmer for about 20 minutes. Cool and strain. Bring to quick boil again, remove from heat immediately, and add 4 ounces of glycerin. Take 1 to 3 tablespoons three to four times daily. Keep the mixture in the refrigerator.

SKULLCAP
Scutellaria laterifolia

OTHER NAMES: Helmet flower, Quaker bonnet, hood-wort, blue pimpernel, American skullcap, blue skullcap, and madweed.
PART USED: The part above ground, gathered while flowering.
SIGNATURE: The bell-shape lid of the calyx suggested to early herbalist that the herb could be used as a treatment for ailments of the skull.

Skullcap has been well known for soothing sleeplessness, headaches, or any nervous disorders. Skullcap contains tannins, glycoside, iron, and vitamin E. It can improve circulation and relieve muscle cramps. This is a good relaxer for those suffering from arthritis since it helps feed and calm the nerves, spinal cord, and brain. This herb is slow-acting. Skullcap requires time to work if it is to be effective; so, you need to take it about a month.

Skullcap acts as an astringent. It contains lignin, glycoside, iron, silicon, and sodium chloride.

To use as a sleep aid for all types of arthritis, prepare this infusion.

SKULLCAP INFUSION

Pour 3 pints of boiling water over 3 ounces of dried skullcap herb. Cover and steep for 30 minutes or until cool. Strain and add 1 pint of honey. Shake well before use. Heat 1 cup before bed to aid sleep.

RASPBERRY
Rubus idaeus

OTHER NAMES: Red raspberry, European raspberry, and American raspberry.

PART USED: Leaves, fruit, and root.
SIGNATURE: Sharp thorns, taste of root, and the red fruit are its signature. The sharp thorns indicate its use to control pain.

Raspberry acts as a diuretic that dispels toxins from the body. The red fruit suggests use as a blood cleanser. And because the root has astringent properties, it has been found to have some antibiotic value because of the high levels of gallic acids and tannic acids. It also contains citric acid, silicon, pectin, and vitamins C and D. Raspberry strengthens the uterine wall, relaxes intestinal spasms, helps heal canker sores, and maintains healthy bones, teeth, skin, and nails.

RASPBERRY VINEGAR

Many old herbals call for use of raspberries in the sick room. To prepare, place red raspberries in a clay or glass container. Cover completely with cider vinegar and allow the mixture to stand overnight, covered. Strain and add 1 pint of sugar to every pint of juice. Boil for ten minutes and place in a sterile jar. To use, place 2 tablespoons of the mixture in 1 glass of ice water. It is very soothing and helpful. Equal parts of black and red raspberries may be used to prepare this mixture.

Caution: Raspberry may inhibit iron absorption.

BUTCHER'S BROOM
Cytisus scoparius

PART USED: The early tops of the branches.
SIGNATURE: It grows in sandy soils near small streams. The ground may even be rocky. The yellow flowers of the plant indicate that it has diuretic properties and can assist in removing kidney stones.

The plant has strong diuretic and laxative action. The herb also contains hydroxytyramine, alkaloids, and ruscogenins. Butcher's broom reduces inflammation. It is good for circulatory disorders, gout, hemorrhoids, jaundice, varicose veins, and leg cramps.

Caution: This herb should be used with caution. If harvested before flowering, it contains spareine, which when taken in large doses can be toxic.

WILLOW
Salix spp.

PART USED: Leaves, twigs, bark, or root.
SIGNATURE: Willows grow around ponds, creeks, lakes, and swamps, and were first considered as a diuretic and febrifuge in feverish colds.

White willow (*Salix alba*) is the tree most often used, although any of the willows has medicinal value. Even the common pussy willow (*Salix caprea*) is frequently prescribed. If used in a natural state, the bark contains salicin and other phytochemicals that enhance the antipyretic, analgesic, antiseptic, and disinfectant properties of the herb.

Salicin and salicylates, originally found in willows, are ingredients in modern aspirin. Willow is frequently prescribed in treatment of arthritis because it reduces inflammation and has pain-relieving properties. The trunk bark is also similar in action to quinine.

WILLOW BARK TEA

To prepare a tea of the willow, place 1 tablespoon of willow bark in 1 pint of cold water. Allow it to soak overnight, covered. Bring to a boil, reduce heat, and simmer for 20 minutes. Strain and refrigerate. Drink about ¼ cup for pain relief.

BURDOCK
Arctium lappa

OTHER NAMES: Lappa, fox's clote, thorny burr, beggar's buttons, love leaves, clotbur, happy major, clothburr, lappa minor, edible burdock.
PART USED: Root, leaves, seed, and stem. But the root is the part used in treatment of arthritis.
SIGNATURE: The round flower head is said to resemble the human head, and the prickles resemble human hair. This suggested use as a preventive of baldness, internally and externally. The color of the stalk is red, which denotes blood-cleansing properties. The seeds indicate the removal of hard stones and treatment of kidney stones.

Burdock can be traced back to ancient times as a medicinal herb. It has been used extensively as a blood cleanser and is one of the ingredients of the Essiac remedy. Essiac is used as a treatment for cancer, AIDS, and as a general tonic for the immune system. It has also been used to treat arthritis and related disorders. It is also known as a memory-enhancing herb.

Burdock is very soothing to mucous membranes all through the body. Burdock contains about 12 percent protein and has about 28 to 45 percent inulin as well as other trace minerals.

BURDOCK DECOCTIONS

You can make a decoction of burdock by adding 2 ounces of the root to 1 pint of water. Bring to a boil and reduce to a simmer for 30 minutes. Strain and drink 1 pint daily if desired. Longtime use is encouraged.

A stronger decoction is 4 ounces of burdock to 2 quarts of water. Soak the roots in the cold water for several hours. Bring to a boil and simmer down to 1 quart. Strain and add 4 ounces of glycerin. Refrigerate. The dosage is from 1 teaspoon up to 1 tablespoon in a small glass of water daily.

ESSIAC

$3^1/_4$ cups of cut burdock root
$^1/_2$ pound of powdered sheep sorrel
$^1/_2$ ounce of powdered turkey rhubarb
2 ounces of slippery elm

Here's the traditional Essiac remedy. Mix the herbs well, and remove $^1/_2$ cup of the herb mixture for immediate use. Keep the remaining mixture in the freezer until needed.

Place $^1/_2$ cup of the herb mixture in 1 gallon of boiling water. Cover and continue boiling for 10 minutes. Remove from heat and allow to stand 12 hours or overnight. Then return the pan to full heat for 20 minutes. Strain and bottle in sterile containers. Refrigerate. The dosage is 2 ounces (4 tablespoons) of the Essiac mixture to 4 tablespoons of water. Drink at least two hours after your evening meal or right before bedtime. This should be taken for an indefinite period of time when treating serious illnesses like cancer or AIDS.

KELP
Fucus vesiculosis

OTHER NAMES: Bladder wrack, black tang, sea-wrack.
SIGNATURE: The swollen glands along the neck of the frond indicates uses for swelling.

It is used as an aid in treating arthritis and goiters. Kelp has blood-cleansing properties and contains iodine, alginic acid, biotin, choline, inositol, bromine, sulfur, calcium, copper, selenium, sodium, potassium, and vitamins A, B_1, B_3, B_5, B_9, B_{12}, C, E, and zinc. It's great for those suffering from mineral deficiencies. It is high in organic iodine plus many other minerals that make it vital to our health. Kelp has the highest amount of trace minerals of any known plant source. All the blood in the circulation system passes through the thyroid gland every 17 minutes. The concentration of iodine present in kelp kills germs; so, it can act as a disinfectant.

Prevention or treatment of arthritis and other related disorders is sometimes accomplished through nutrition. When acid-producing foods are eaten, some people suffer painful episodes, such as gout attacks, due to the buildup of uric acids. Lack of essential minerals and vitamins leads to irritation of the nerves and their myelin sheaths. This causes inflammation and swelling. Iodine can interrupt this chain to pain.

Herbalists suggest 8 tablets daily.

SASSAFRAS
Sassafras albidum (Sassafras varifolium)

OTHER NAMES: Gumbo, mitten tree, saloop, auge tree, cinnamon wood, laurus sassafras, saxifrax, and salap.
PART USED: Leaves and root bark.
SIGNATURE: The tree seems to sprout from between the crevices or clefts of rocks. Thus, breaking through hard substances would be its signature.

Sassafras is a wonderful blood cleanser and removes obstructions from mucous linings. It contains many minerals, including zinc, manganese, sulfur, sodium, and sarsaponin as well as vitamins A and D. Sassafras was declared a wonder drug during the 16th century. It is still used today to fortify and thin the blood and has a high mineral content.

An interesting side note: Add a handful of sassafras to dried fruit to keep insects away.

You can make stimulating liniment by mixing equal parts of oil of sassafras, oil of cloves, and oil of cinnamon.

To make an infusion to drink, pour 1 pint of boiling water over 1 ounce of crushed or chipped sassafras. Cover and steep 10 minutes. Strain and drink daily if desired.

VIOLET
Viola odorata

PART USED: Leaves and flowers.
SIGNATURE: The signature is the glutinous taste. Violet has expectorant and emollient properties.

There are about 400 different varieties of violet. The plant contains glucosides with antiseptic properties that reach where only blood and lymphatic fluids can penetrate. Violet is high in vitamin A, and a rich source of vitamin A is essential for treating inflammations. The vitamin is also essential for keeping joints limber, soft, and pliable.

You can powder the herb and use it in capsule form or prepare it as a tea to help relieve the inflammation of arthritis. Use fresh or dried leaves and flowers. If using fresh, add 1 tablespoon of the chopped herb to 1 cup of boiling water. Cover and steep for 10 minutes. Strain, add honey if desired, and drink daily. If using the dried herb, add only 1 teaspoon of the herb to the boiling water.

BLACK COHOSH
Cimicifuga racemosa

OTHER NAMES: Squawroot, black snakeroot, rattleweed, rattleroot, bugbane.
PART USED: Root and rhizomes.

Black cohosh contains magnesium, phosphorus, potassium, salts, silicon, and vitamins B_3, B_5, B_9, E, and A. While it has many wonderful properties, its ability to reduce inflammation is why it is favored in treatment of arthritis. Black cohosh also exerts a tonic influence over serous tissue and mucous membranes due to the magnesium phosphate it contains. It has long been a favorite of Native Americans as a treatment for arthritis and rheumatism. Black cohosh is a nerve and muscle relaxant.

The herb can be used as a tincture or powdered in capsules or combined with other herbs. The oil can be extracted only in alcohol. You can add the tincture to teas, juices, or water to be taken daily. Here's how to make the tincture.

BLACK COHOSH TINCTURE

Put 1 ounce of the black cohosh root into a quart jar. Cover the herb completely with vodka or brandy, and place in a warm, preferably sunny, area for about two weeks. Shake daily. Strain and bottle. The dosage is $1/2$ to 1 full dropper of the tincture in juice, water, or tea.

SLIPPERY ELM
Ulmus fulvus

OTHER NAMES: Moose elm, American elm, red elm, Indian elm.
PART USED: The dried inner bark.
SIGNATURE: You can tell what the signature is after chewing on the bark. It has a sweetish taste and is very mucilaginous. The properties of the bark are emollient and demulcent.

The bark contains bioflavonoids and vitamin K along with calcium, phosphorus, tannins, polysaccharides, and starch. It can be used as a food as well as a medicine. Early settlers and Native Americans ate the gruel from slippery elm when food supplies were low or gone, because the herb was available year-round and (we've discovered) has high nutritive value.

SLIPPERY ELM GRUEL

To prepare the gruel, simply add 1 teaspoon of slippery elm to 1 teaspoon of cold water or milk. Then add an additional 1 pint of hot water or milk, stirring continuously. Lemon or cinnamon may be added as flavoring, if desired. In earlier centuries European children who were weaned were also given a gruel as a nutritive aid. Add 1 tablespoon slippery elm to 1 teaspoon of cold water. Then stir this mixture into 1 pint of hot milk.

Slippery elm provides nutritive support for cartilage, bones, and affected tissue. This is why Native Americans have continued to use it to help relieve arthritis and rheumatism. It can be used in any condition involving inflamed or injured tissue or bone. It is very soothing to the mucous membranes of the stomach, bowel, and urinary tract. In fact, slippery elm has cleansing, soothing, and healing properties beneficial to the whole body.

SLIPPERY ELM TEA

You can make a tea by adding 1 teaspoon of slippery elm to 1 cup of boiling water. Steep at least an hour. Strain and reheat. This thick tea will have the consistency of syrup. Drink as often as desired.

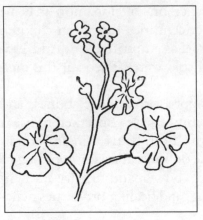

Cranesbill

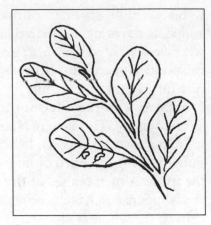

Sumac

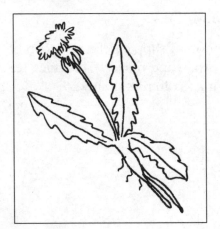

Dandelion

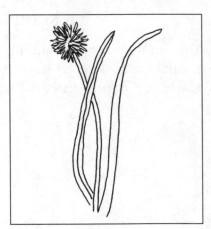

Garlic

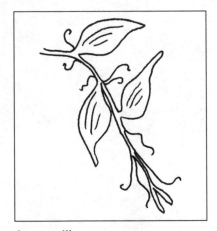

Sarsaparilla

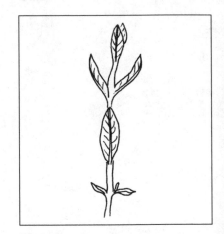

Bitter Root

2. Diabetes Mellitus

Of all the serious diseases that afflict humankind, diabetes is perhaps the most easily controlled through diet.

Diabetes symptoms were first described in medical documents dating from 1500 B.C. Proper treatment was then unknown, and it was not until the 19th century that sugar in the urine was related to an abnormality of the pancreas.

Only recently have indigenous people on continents other than Eurasia and Africa begun to suffer from this disorder. When these peoples changed from their natural diet to a European refined diet, they began to acquire diabetes. Today, many herbalists and nutritionists believe that a return to an improved, natural diet would halt this insidious epidemic.

One out of twenty Americans has diabetes. Another 20 million suffer from it but are unaware that they have it. And yet another 20 million have glucose intolerance that could lead to full-blown diabetes. Diabetes is the fourth leading cause of death in the United States. It is also the leading cause of kidney disorders, blindness, amputation, and impotence. People with diabetes have a two to six times greater chance of having a heart attack or stroke than the rest of the population.

Type I (juvenile) diabetes is caused by destruction of the body's insulin-producing cells. Diabetes results from production of insufficient amounts of insulin by the pancreas.

Type II (adult-onset) diabetes has many causes and can be more easily controlled through changed lifestyle. A natural diet, with more whole foods and fewer processed foods, lowers the body's need for insulin and helps reduce the complications of diabetes. Age, weight, and heredity also influence type II diabetes.

Nearly all people with type II diabetes are able to produce insulin. However, the body is unable to use it properly. Weight loss and a daily exercise program can help control this disorder. Realizing that diabetes is a chronic illness may help explain its seriousness.

Insulin is a hormone that helps the body use energy created by starches, sugars, and other foods. Glucose, a source of energy for the body and brain, is a sugar produced when the body digests sugar, starches, and carbohydrates. It is the body's major source of fuel for the energy it needs. Without insulin, blood sugar (blood glucose) levels increase. And these high blood glucose levels can lead to both short- and long-term problems.

Although anyone can get diabetes, people of Hispanic, American Indian, or African descent are at greater risk. People over 40, with a family history of diabetes, and who are overweight or who have had a baby weighing more than 9 pounds, are at risk of acquiring diabetes.

Type I (juvenile) diabetes symptoms include these four things: (1) frequent urination, (2) extreme thirst and hunger, (3) weakness and tiredness, and (4) weight loss. People with this chronic disorder are insulin-dependent. Type I, insulin-dependent, diabetes must be monitored by a physician. Talk with a diabetes educator, physician, or nurse about diet and management.

About 90 percent of people with diabetes have adult-onset, type II diabetes. It usually takes many years to develop this type. Most people with this disorder are over 40. This type of diabetes is more easily controlled with a change in diet. And weight loss may be the single most important controlling factor for type II diabetes.

Type II (adult-onset) diabetes symptoms are these: (1) blurred vision, (2) loss of feeling in hands and feet, (3) dry, itchy skin, (4) extreme tiredness, (5) bladder infections and skin rashes, (6) frequent urination, (7) vaginal yeast infections, (8) lingering flu-like symptoms, (9) hair loss on legs, (10) increased facial hair, (11) xanthomas—small yellow bumps of fat and cholesterol under the skin, and (12) inflammation of penile skin.

Often no symptoms are present when diabetes is diagnosed from the presence of sugar in the urine. Adult-onset diabetes is often associated with arteriosclerosis. Most common infections involve the gums, skin, bladder, vagina, and lungs, often resulting in bronchitis and pneumonia. People with diabetes who do not control their blood glucose have difficulty fighting infections. They also suffer from these disorders more frequently than the rest of the population.

Gestational diabetes is developed during pregnancy. Two to 3 percent of all pregnant women develop gestational diabetes. Again, women who are over 40 and overweight are the most likely candidates. Gestational diabetes is more common in American Indian, African, and Hispanic women than in the general population. Of this 2 to 3 percent, about 35 percent will develop type II diabetes at a later date.

Because diet can help control both weight and diabetes, it is important to learn about the foods you should and should not eat. There are two forms of carbohydrates, simple and complex. Simple carbohydrates include fruits, fruit juices, vegetables, honey, jellies, candies, and desserts. Complex carbohydrates include starchy foods like bread, rice, pasta, cereal, grains, and starchy vegetables. Foods high in complex carbohydrates should provide 50 to 60 percent of your daily calories. Eat larger amounts of starchy foods and fewer high-fat or high-protein foods. Avoid refined carbohydrates—processed breads and cereals from which much of the nutrition has been lost.

Proteins help build tissue and act as energy reserves. Meat, fish, poultry, cheese, eggs, milk, dried beans, legumes, and some nuts are good sources of protein. But high-fat protein sources should be avoided. Protein should make up 12 to 20 percent of your daily calories. You can get this amount from two small portions daily.

Fat is stored in the body as extra calories for future use. Fats are found in margarine, butter, oils, nuts, meat, and dairy products like ice cream or milk. Limit the high-fat foods you eat. Saturated fats should make up less than 10 percent of your daily calories. Total fats should make up no more than 30 percent of your daily total calories.

A high-fiber and high-carbohydrate diet reduces the need for insulin and lowers blood-sugar surges, as well as fat levels in the blood.

Along with these dietary restrictions, people with diabetes need to reduce stress in their lives and increase daily exercise. Vitamin and mineral supplements help treat diabetes. At least 17 vitamins, 20 minerals, and 16 amino acids are thought essential to good health. This is true for everyone, not just people with diabetes.

Insulin cannot function without *chromium,* and it may be that many people with diabetes are suffering from a chromium deficiency. In the early stages of type II diabetes, it has been suggested that the disease could be reversed with a chromium supplement. According to an April 1966 report by the U.S. Federal Drug Administration (FDA), a group of infant refugees in Jerusalem were treated by a local pediatrician and a U.S. FDA scientist. These children were all severely malnourished and most had faulty glucose metabolism. They were given a small amount of chromium in their daily diet, and all made "overnight" recoveries from the body's inability to use sugar.

RECOMMENDED NUTRIENTS

Just 200 mcg of *chromium* daily helps stabilize blood sugar and increase energy. Chromium deficiency is much more prevalent in Western countries than in Africa, the Middle East, or the Far East because people in these areas do not eat as many refined foods.

Good sources of chromium are whole grains and seeds. The chromium in wheat germ is concentrated in the germ. Adding wheat germ to your daily diet helps provide protection. Brewer's yeast has the highest amount of chromium of any natural source. Next is black pepper, then calves' liver, American cheese, wheat germ, eggs, and oysters.

In clinical trials 50 percent of patients with abnormal blood glucose levels had blood glucose levels restored to normal on a daily dose of 150 mcg of trivalent chromium, found in brewer's yeast. Twelve older patients also took brewer's yeast on a trial basis, and half of them regained the body's ability to metabolize blood sugar within two months. Brewer's yeast also lowers the insulin requirements of some insulin-dependent diabetics.

Only 10 percent of people with diabetes have insufficient insulin production. The other 90 percent of diabetes cases are not caused by lack of insulin, but by a condition called insulin-resistance. In other words, the pancreas produces insulin, but the insulin just does not work. The trace element *vanadium* works like oral insulin or better, according to Julian Whittaker, M.D., editor of the magazine *Health and Healing*. In experiments with animals, sufficient doses of vanadyl sulfate, a form of vanadium, were given with the result that the diabetes was completely reversed and did not come back.

Dr. Whittaker has recommended that his patients take 100 to 150 mcg per day, in divided doses with meals. He also recommends a low-fat diet and a supplement of chromium picolinate and magnesium. For some of his patients, diabetes has been reversed, and it appears to be a permanent result. Vanadyl sulfate can be bought at health food stores. This supplement may cause some gastrointestinal disturbance. If so, reduce or stop the supplement and then start over, slowly increasing the dosage.

Other recommended nutrients for people with diabetes are magnesium; calcium; vitamins A, C, and E; and apple pectin.

Magnesium is important for pH balance and the enzyme system. Usually 750 mg daily is recommended.

Calcium is also needed for pH balance, with 1500 mg suggested daily.

Also, take 15,000 IU of *vitamin A* daily, but avoid taking beta-carotene supplements, since people with diabetes cannot convert it into vitamin A. Cod liver oil is a good vitamin A source.

Vitamin E is important to prevent vascular damage. *Vitamin C* is also important. In 1974, George V. Mann, M.D., in *Perspectives in Biology and Medicine* stated that lesions that develop and impede the circulation of blood vessels in patients with diabetes are a form of scurvy, or vitamin C deficiency. Linus Pauling, M.D., also confirms these results. In the *Journal of Applied Nutrition* in 1972, Fred R. Klenner, M.D., stated that patients who received 10 grams daily of vitamin C normalized healing of wounds. And they were able to make better use of insulin, so they required less.

Apple pectin is very good for diabetes. It slows the absorption of foods and removes toxins and undesirable metals from the body. Pectin can be used as a sugar substitute. It is found in apples, bananas, citrus fruits, peas, carrots, beets, and cabbage.

If you have diabetes, add these foods to your daily diet to help normalize blood sugar.

FOODS THAT NORMALIZE BLOOD SUGAR

Berries	Egg Yolks	String Beans	Fruit Juices
Brewer's Yeast	Garlic	Whole Grains	Oats
Dairy Products	Fish	Seeds	Beans
Nuts	Spinach	Fruits	Soybeans
Sauerkraut	Broccoli	Honey	Raw Vegetables
Cucumber	Red Currant	American	Jerusalem
Juice	Juice	Cheese	Artichokes
Onions	Cabbage	Melons	Squashes
Asparagus	Celery	Oils	Cereals

Most of the proteins and salts you digest should come from vegetable sources. All plants contain chlorine in the form of sodium chloride.

Soybeans, a good food source, are made up of 40 percent protein, 20 percent fat, and 2 percent lecithin. They also contain steroidsaponine and vitamins B_1, B_2, E, and provitamin-A. One cup of cooked soybeans contains about the same number of calories (298 calories) and the same number of grams of protein (28 g) as 4 ounces of lean beef. Dried kidney bean pods can be made into a strong decoction that, when used as a diuretic, helps lower blood sugar.

Whole grains and seeds aid in slowing the absorption of sugar into the blood. Unrefined rolled oats contain calcium and a large variety of minerals. Cereals and goat's milk are also helpful.

Cucumber juice and cucumbers help lower blood sugar. Jerusalem artichokes contain inulin and levulin. These carbohydrates are not converted into sugar in the body. Jerusalem artichokes are high in vitamins and minerals and can be eaten raw, boiled, baked, or pickled and used in stews, soups, and salads.

HELPFUL HERBS

Humans have used herbs for millennia. The herbs listed here as helpful for people with diabetes is small, but many more herbs could be useful. These recommended herbs are sumac, alum root, bearberry, saw palmetto, ginseng, dandelion, prickly ash bark, bilberry, cranesbill, black walnut, sarsaparilla, bitter root, kelp, and garlic. See chapter 10 for more botanical sources of minerals, vitamins, and trace elements.

SUMAC
Rhus glabra

OTHER NAMES: Indian salt, scarlet sumac, dwarf sumac, smooth sumac, vinegar tree.
PART USED: Berries and bark.
SIGNATURE: The red fruit, round bark openings, and the velvety hairs covering the stems and trunk of the plant are its signature.

SUMAC BERRY–BLUEBERRY TEA

This old remedy combines sumac berries with blueberries. Cover the berries completely with boiling water. Remove from heat and cover.

Steep for 1 to 2 hours. Strain and measure the juice; add an equal amount of honey. Bring to a boil and cook 10 to 15 minutes. Pour the resulting syrup into a sterile container and seal. Add 1 teaspoon of syrup to 1 cup boiling water. Drink twice daily.

ALUM ROOT
Heuchera americana

OTHER NAMES: American sanicle, wild geranium, rock geranium.
PART USED: Root.

Alum root contains potassium, so it would be good to add to your daily diet. It acts as an astringent and diuretic. Add $^1/_4$ teaspoon of dried powdered alum root to 1 cup of water. Drink $^1/_3$ cup three times daily for three to four days per week.

BEARBERRY
Arctostaphylos uva-ursi

OTHER NAMES: Upland cranberry, mountain cranberry, uva ursi, mountain box, bear's grape, rockberry, sandberry, mealberry, creashak.
PART USED: Fruit and evergreen leaves.
SIGNATURE: Red berries, found growing over rocky, sandy, or gravely areas, are its signature.

Bearberry possesses diuretic and antiseptic properties. It is helpful in diabetes for reducing excessive blood sugar levels and for treating pancreatic disorders.

BEARBERRY TINCTURE or TEA

Make a tincture by placing the leaves of the bearberry in a quart jar and tightly pack down and cover the herb completeiy with vodka or brandy. Cover and allow the mixture to stand in a warm area or sunny window for two weeks. You can mix blueberry leaves with bearberry leaves, half and half, if desired. This makes the tincture more effective. Take 10 to 20 drops of tincture three to four times daily. To use as a tea, place 1 teaspoon of the soaked leaves in a cup. Pour 1 cup of boiling water over the leaves. Cover and allow the mixture to steep 15 minutes. Strain and drink 2 to 3 cups daily.

SAW PALMETTO
Serenoa serrulata

OTHER NAMES: Fan palm, sabal, dwarf palmetto.
PART USED: Berries.

Saw palmetto contains volatile oils, alkaloid, resin, dextrin, and glucose. It has an effect on all glands and is helpful for kidney disorders and diabetes.

SAW PALMETTO TINCTURE

You can prepare saw palmetto as a tincture or use it as a tea. To prepare the tea, simply place 1 teaspoon of the berries in a cup. Pour 1 cup of boiling water over the berries and cover. Steep 15 minutes. Strain and drink. To prepare a tincture, place the berries in a jar; cover completely with vodka or brandy. Put on a tight lid and place the jar in a warm area or sunny window. Allow it to steep for two weeks, shaking occasionally. Strain and bottle in a sterile container for future use. Place 1 teaspoon of the tincture in 1 cup of boiling water. Drink daily if desired.

GINSENG
Panax quinquefolius

OTHER NAMES: Root of life, root of man, seed of earth, panacea, life everlasting, American ginseng, sang, five-finger root, panex, santa root, ninsin, pannag, red berry, man's health.
PART USED: The dried leaves and root.
SIGNATURE: The root resembles a human shape.

It arouses the lymphatic glands, stimulates blood circulation, increases capillary circulation in the brain, and activates the metabolism and the kidneys.

To prepare a tea of the leaves, add 1 teaspoon of the leaves to 1 cup of boiling water. Cover and steep 15 minutes. Strain and drink.

Another way to prepare the tea is to mix 6 ounces of the powdered root with 2 ounces of honey and 60 drops of wintergreen. Mix well. Add 1 teaspoon of the mixture to 1 cup of boiling water. Steep covered 10 to 15 minutes. You can drink several cups per day as long as desired.

DANDELION
Taraxacum officinale (Leontodon taraxacum)

OTHER NAMES: Blow ball, lion's tooth, wild endive, cankerwort.
PART USED: Virtually all the plant is used, but the root is more commonly favored for medicinal purposes.
SIGNATURE: The yellow flowers are its signature.

The leaves contain 7,000 IU of vitamin A per ounce, along with vitamins B complex and C, bioflavonoids, PABA, sulfur, biotin, zinc, iron, phosphorus, and more. The plant makes a wonderful tonic for the liver. Dandelion also contains 28 parts sodium, which is a good type of natural nutritive salt. It destroys acids in the blood and purifies the blood. It contains inulin.

You can use the leaves as a salad green or as a cooked green. Add the flowers along with the greens to soups or stews. Add the dried root to coffee. The powdered root can be taken in capsule form or added to other teas. Use 1 teaspoon per cup of boiling water along with other herbs. Eat as much of the greens as desired, and the tea can be drunk daily.

PRICKLY ASH BARK
Zanthoxylum americanum

OTHER NAMES: Toothache tree, suterberry, yellow wood, northern prickly ash.
PART USED: Bark.
SIGNATURE: The yellow inner bark is its signature.

This herb is helpful when the liver and pancreas are not functioning well.

PRICKLY ASH TEA

Prickly ash bark is used as a tea. Add 1 teaspoon of the bark to 1 cup of boiling water. Cover and steep 15 minutes. Strain and drink. Prepare just 1 cup of tea, and drink it throughout the day.

BILBERRY
Vaccinium myrtillus

OTHER NAMES: High bush, swamp blueberry, whortleberry, whinberry, hurtleberry, huckleberry.
PART USED: Leaves and berries.
SIGNATURE: The signature is that the berries contain many seeds, and the plant is found in swampy areas.

BILBERRY TINCTURE

Prepare a tincture by placing 2 ounces of bilberry leaves and/or berries in a jar with 1 quart of vodka or brandy. Cover and place in a warm or sunny window, shaking daily for four weeks. Strain and pour the liquid into a sterile container and seal. Add 1 to 2 teaspoons of the tincture to 1 cup of boiling water. Drink three to four times daily.

Scientists from the former Soviet Union had established that bilberry is similar to insulin. And we now know that bilberry helps promote insulin production.

CRANESBILL
Geranium maculatum

OTHER NAMES: Dovesfoot, alum root, wild geranium, wild cranesbill, spotted geranium, crowfoot, American kino.
PART USED: Dried root and leaves.
SIGNATURE: The red hue from the fading leaves is cranesbill's signature.

CRANESBILL TEA

Mix 3 tablespoons of oak bark, 1 tablespoon of cranesbill, 1 tablespoon of sumac berries, and 1 tablespoon of witch hazel leaves. Add 1 tablespoon of this mixture to 1 quart of boiling water. Boil gently for 20 minutes, remove from heat, cover, and cool. Strain when the tea is cool and bottle in a sterile container. Drink $1/3$ cup of tea daily.

BLACK WALNUT
Juglans nigra

PART USED: Bark, leaves, rind, and green nut.
SIGNATURE: The nuts are shaped like the human head. The gray and black fissures on the trunk of the tree and the astringency of the leaves are also its signature.

Herbalists have long prescribed the leaves of three herbs to help lower blood sugar: walnut, avocado, and eucalyptus.

TEAS FOR LOWERING BLOOD SUGAR

Try a tea made of walnut leaves in the morning. Add 1 teaspoon of fresh or dried walnut leaves to 1 cup of boiling water. Steep 15 minutes, strain, and drink.

In the afternoon, try a tea made of avocado leaves. Make it the same way as the walnut-leaf tea.

And at night, try a tea made from eucalyptus leaves. Continue this regimen until the urine is sugar-free.

SARSAPARILLA
Aralia nudicaulis

OTHER NAMES: Small spikenard, spignet, red sarsaparilla, wild sarsaparilla, quill, quay.
PART USED: Root.
SIGNATURE: Sarsaparilla is a member of the ginseng family (*Araliaceae*), so that suggests it would promote blood purification. It also has long roots with a creeping pattern.

Sarsaparilla contains potassium chloride, basserin, albumen, pectin and acetic acid, essential oils, magnesium, lime, salts of potash, and iron oxide. Sarsaparilla eliminates poisons from the blood and purifies the body. Prepare as a tea or beverage. Take as much as desired daily.

BITTER ROOT
Apocynum androsaemifolium

OTHER NAMES: Milk weed, westerwall, common dogbane, spreading dogbane.
PART USED: All parts, but the root is preferred.
SIGNATURE: The milk of the plant resembles mother's milk and was once used to treat faulty lactation.

BITTER ROOT SYRUP

Prepare a syrup by macerating the roots and placing them in a pan. Cover the roots completely with boiling water. Bring to a boil again, then reduce heat, and simmer for 30 minutes, covered. Remove from heat and allow the mixture to stand at least an hour. Strain and measure. Add an equal amount of honey. Pour into a sterile container and seal. Add 1 teaspoon of the mixture to 1 cup of boiling water. Drink 1 cup daily. Bitter root is a good tonic for the whole immune system.

KELP
Fucus vesiculosis

OTHER NAMES: Bladder wrack, sea wrack, black tang.

The most important minerals needed for the body are iodine, calcium, phosphorus, manganese, sodium, potassium, magnesium, chlorine, and sulfur. Because our overworked soils are almost depleted of these minerals needed to maintain health, we have begun to turn to the sea. Oceans are rich in vital minerals. Because the blood has a composition similar to that of sea water, it makes sense to supply our mineral needs with kelp, a vegetable from the sea. We know that plants are the only living organisms capable of manufacturing food.

Kelp contains most of the minerals we need to sustain life. Calcium, phosphorus, magnesium, sodium, potassium, chlorine, sulfur, iron, iodine, strontium, silicon, manganese, copper, tin, lead, vanadium, zinc, titanium, chromium, barium, and silver are in kelp. It is also a good source of biotin, PABA, and vitamins A, E, B complex, D, and E. Kelp also contains mannitol, which is a bile stimulant; a phosphorous compound that helps to knit broken bones; and small amounts of lecithin.

Herbalists recommend as many as 8 kelp tablets daily.

GARLIC
Allium sativum or *Allium canadense*

OTHER NAMES: Wild garlic, meadow leek, rose leek, wild onion.
PART USED: Leaves and bulbs.
SIGNATURE: The leaves are long and tubular. The urinary systems are hollow, so the signature of garlic suggests its use in the urinary system.

Garlic prevents infections. An equal mixture of garlic and onions, cooked together, has been found to be as good as tolbutamide, a standard drug used in treatment of diabetes. Include both in your daily diet as often as possible. Garlic also lowers high blood pressure. Insufficient insulin, the hormone associated with diabetes, is always associated with high blood pressure.

BREWER'S YEAST
Brewer's yeast should be added to your daily diet along with potassium, zinc, chromium, manganese, calcium, and magnesium. Brewer's yeast is rich in all the B-complex vitamins, except B_{12}. A vitamin B_6 deficiency can induce abnormal glucose tolerance, similar to that of diabetes.

Present in brewer's yeast are sixteen amino acids, fourteen or more minerals, and seventeen vitamins. Protein makes up 52 percent of its weight. Since it is high in phosphorus, you need to take calcium with it. The source of brewer's yeast is hops. All plants contain vitamins and minerals we need to sustain health. Hops is but one example that contains many of these nutrients.

Brewer's yeast has many times higher amounts of chromium than any other food. It has been estimated that half of all diabetes cases may have been induced by a chromium-deficient diet. Mother Nature has supplied the body with the insulin needed, but this hormone, like others in the body, cannot do the job alone. We need the proper fuel in order to ensure that the whole engine receives the nutrients we need and should be getting from a natural diet. Brewer's yeast is the best source of the biologically available chromium that we all need.

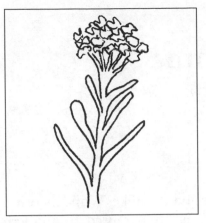

Pleurisy Root

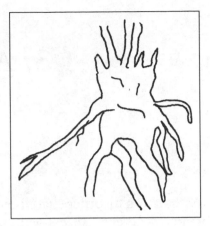

Elecampane

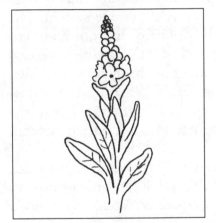

Mullein

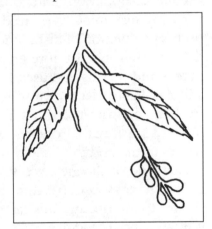

Wild Cherry

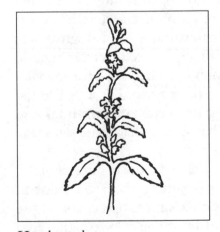

Horehound

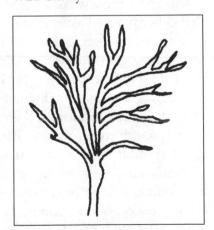

Ephedra

3. Asthma

Asthma is a disorder shared by young and old alike. While there are many different causes, asthma today is often caused by modern chemicals, pollution, and food allergies. An attack is usually triggered by histamine, produced by the body's immune system. The body's production of histamine is its way of providing antibodies to defend itself against foreign invaders. But this can cause excess mucus and spasms in muscles surrounding the bronchi, which then affect and constrict the outward passage of air. When air cannot pass freely to or from the small air sacs within the lungs, the result is bronchial asthma. Bronchial asthma may also be caused by acid wastes in the body.

Any kind of allergic reaction can cause the immune system to kick in, which may cause an asthma attack. Often children with asthma are allergic to aspirin, and this can provoke an attack, as can tartrazino, a yellow artificial food dye (yellow #5).

Cardiac asthma is caused by a malfunctioning heart. Research shows that other types of asthma may be the result of magnesium deficiency.

Vitamin B_6 (pyridoxine) has been demonstrated to be of great help in preventing asthma attacks. Those who respond to this treatment do not have a deficiency, they just have an exaggerated need for the vitamin because of disturbed metabolism. The suggested dose is 100 mg of B_6 daily for one month, then 200 mg the second month. It takes at least a month to get results. Research has shown that those who take 200 mg suffer fewer severe asthma attacks.

Symptoms are easy to recognize. Onset can be sudden, often at night. The asthma sufferer has intense difficulty breathing, the face is pale and the expression often anxious. The person feels great oppression in the chest, fears suffocation, and has labored breathing. Dry cough, rapid pulse, sweating, coldness of extremities, and drowsiness often occur.

Asthmatic children use up their blood sugar fast, so it's advisable to give them orange juice with honey added, morning and evening. Restrict the use of sugar and substitute honey in their diet.

Nature holds many cures. Often herbs are used in a steam or burned for inhalation. The vapor of the oils released is taken into the lungs and absorbed by the whole body.

In India, the *Tylophora indica* plant leaves are used in the treatment of asthma. The patient is given a single leaf to chew every day for one week. After this treatment, the asthma is said to be suppressed for up to three months.

Garlic syrup is often used in treatment of asthma. Place one pound of chopped, fresh garlic in a stainless-steel container, and pour 1 quart of boiling water over the garlic. Cover tightly and allow it to stand overnight. Boil 1 tablespoon of bruised caraway and 1 tablespoon of fennel seed in 3 tablespoons of apple cider vinegar for a short period of time. Strain and add to the strained garlic water. Measure the liquid and add an equal amount of honey. Take several tablespoons daily as a preventative and treatment.

Castor oil (*Ricinus communis*) or palm of Christ (*Palma Christi*) packs are often used to treat asthma. Place a flannel cloth in a cake pan and saturate it with cold-pressed castor oil. Place the pan in a warm oven long enough to heat the cloth. You do not want the cloth to get too hot, just warm. Place the warmed flannel cloth on the back and kidney area, covering as much as possible. Lay a large plastic bag or plastic wrap over the cloth, and cover that with a heating pad. Cover the back with a heavy towel or blanket, and allow the treatment to continue for at least an hour daily several times a week. You can then place the cloth back in the pan, and store it in a plastic bag for future use.

The diet should include plenty of fresh vegetables and fruits. Fasting once a month using distilled water and lemon juice seems to be helpful in flushing toxins and mucus from the body. Avoid sulfites in your diet. They are commonly used in restaurants to preserve raw fruits and vegetables in salad bars, and they are included in many other foods from the grocery store. If you or your children suffer from asthma, you might consider getting test strips that detect the presence of sulfites in foods. Better yet, consider growing and preserving your own foods. You'll then know that your produce is fresh and without additives.

RECOMMENDED NUTRIENTS

If you have asthma, it is important to eat foods and ingest herbs that contain *copper, manganese, magnesium,* and *iron,* as well as *vitamins B_6, C,* and *E.* Turn to chapter 10 and choose an herb from each nutrient group recommended and mix them together. Add 1 teaspoon of the herb mixture to 1 cup of boiling water, and steep covered for 15 minutes. Strain, sweeten with honey, and drink a cup with each meal. Change your herb selections frequently so that you will be able to maintain this regimen.

Be sure to include foods from the recommended nutrient lists in your daily diet.

HELPFUL HERBS

Also, these special herbs may be helpful for asthma: juniper berries, licorice root, slippery elm, ephedra (take with great caution), wild cherry bark, mullein, horehound, pleurisy root, elecampane, skunk cabbage, elder flowers and berries, and lobelia. Included here are recipes for teas, tinctures, infusions, and other remedies with descriptions of these herbs.

JUNIPER BERRIES
Juniperus communis

OTHER NAMES: Juniper bush, common juniper, horse-savin' berries.
PART USED: The dried berries.
SIGNATURE: Juniper grows in dry or limestone hills with sand and stone in the area. It was once thought that juniper would remove hardened mucus.

Juniper was once used extensively and revered by ancient Egyptians. Today, it is counted among our most valuable and useful herbs.

Juniper berries remove catarrhal deposits from the whole body. Since the berries are used to clean the body, this makes them valuable for treating asthma.

Juniper contains alcohols, volatile oils, resin, sugar, cadinene, sabinal, tannins, sulfur, camphene, and terpinene, which make it useful in treatment of asthma.

Caution: Juniper berries can interfere with the absorption of iron and other minerals.

JUNIPER BERRY INFUSION, TEA, OR TINCTURE

You can prepare an infusion by mashing about 4 tablespoons of the dried berries and allowing them to soak in 1 quart of boiling water for 1 hour. Strain and drink $\frac{1}{2}$ cup throughout the day until it's gone. Prepare the infusion fresh daily.

You can make a tea one cup at a time from 1 teaspoon of crushed, dried juniper berries added to 1 cup of boiling water. Cover and steep 15 minutes. Strain and drink three times daily.

If you prefer, you can chew the berries, three to four at a time. For a tincture, mash the berries and place them in a quart jar. Cover completely with brandy or vodka. Place the jar in a warm area or sunny window for several weeks, shaking daily. Strain and place the mixture in a sterile bottle. Take 1 tablespoon of the tincture in juice, tea, or boiling water. Children should use only 1 teaspoon of the tincture to 1 cup of liquid.

LICORICE ROOT
Glycyrrhiza glabra

OTHER NAMES: Sweetwood, Spanish juice root, Italian root, liquorice.
PART USED: Root.
SIGNATURE: The long root is sweet and has mucilaginous properties.

Licorice root has antiinflammatory and antitussive properties. It relieves inflammations of the respiratory system. Studies have shown that licorice root is as effective as codeine for suppressing coughs. A hormone found in the root is useful for treatment of asthma.

Licorice root contains PABA, pantothenic acid, and vitamins B_1, B_2, B_3, B_5, B_6, B_9, and E. It also contains the minerals manganese and phosphorus as well as protein, sugar, biotin, choline, inositol, and lecithin.

The use of licorice root promotes the production of interferon, aids adrenal gland function, decreases muscles spasms, and increases the fluidity of mucus from bronchial tubes and lungs. It also reduces stress.

Caution: Avoid use of licorice root if you have high blood pressure or cardiovascular disease.

LICORICE ROOT DECOCTIONS

For a decoction, add 2 ounces of cut licorice root to 2 pints of cold water. Allow the mixture to stand at least several hours. Bring to a boil using a very low heat. Then, simmer gently for about 15 minutes. Strain and add 1 pint of honey. Bring to a boil again; then remove from heat. Cool and bottle. The dosage is 1 to 2 tablespoons as needed every three to four hours.

You can also make another decoction by mixing 2 tablespoons each of licorice root, marshmallow root, pleurisy root, and ¹/₂ ounce of Irish moss. Simmer the herb mixture, covered, in 2 quarts of water. Strain and add 2 ounces of honey. The dosage is ¹/₂ cup four times daily.

SLIPPERY ELM BARK
Ulmus rubra (Ulmus fulva)

OTHER NAMES: Red elm, American elm, moose elm, Indian elm.
PART USED: Dried inner bark.
SIGNATURE: The bark, when chewed, yields a bland mucilaginous substance.

The mucilaginous substance makes slippery elm valuable as a demulcent and emollient. It is a mild expectorant that helps remove phlegm from the bronchial system. The inner bark contains calcium, phosphorus, starch, mucilage, tannins, polysaccharides, bioflavonoids, and vitamin K.

Its uses are many. Slippery elm, combined with elecampane, is used to treat scours (diarrhea or dysentery) in calves. The leaves and twigs, which have a nutty taste, can be chewed to relieve hunger for long periods of time. Slippery elm has the same nutritive value as oatmeal and can be eaten as a gruel. It can also be used alone or mixed with other herbs.

SLIPPERY ELM SYRUP

Place 2 teaspoons of slippery elm bark in 2 pints of water and allow the mixture to stand overnight. Bring to a low boil the next morning and simmer for 15 to 20 minutes. Strain and store. This makes a thick syrup that can be taken by the teaspoon every hour. It soothes and lines the bronchial system, and it also helps remove phlegm.

EPHEDRA
Ephedra sinica, Ephedra nevadensis, Ephedra viridis

OTHER NAMES: Mormon valley plant, desert tea, teamster's tea, ma huang.
PART USED: Top. *Use this herb with extreme caution.*
SIGNATURE: Perhaps the signature of ephedra is that it grows in dry, warm areas.

The ephedra plant has been used for over 4,000 years. It is the source of ephedrine, found in many over-the-counter cold, cough, and asthma medicines as well as in many prescription drugs. But ephedra must be used with caution and under a physician's guidance.

Caution: Ephedra causes constriction of blood vessels and widening of bronchial passages. So, it should not be used by people with high blood pressure or with heart conditions. Also, people who have anxiety attacks or glaucoma should avoid it. Monoamine oxidase inhibitor drugs (commonly prescribed for depression) also should not be used with ephedra.

This bronchodilator is often used in treating asthma. Ephedra speeds up metabolism and has been added to some weight-reduction formulas, but often in dangerously high amounts. It can exhaust the adrenal glands when used for long periods or in a high dosage. It should only be taken for acute asthmatic episodes. Seek a physician's care in use of this herb.

EPHEDRA TEA

You can prepare a tea using twigs of the ephedra plant. Simmer 1 teaspoon of chopped twigs of ephedra along with 2 to 3 teaspoons of schizandra berries in 1 cup of boiling water, covered, for about 10 minutes. Strain and add 1 teaspoon of ginger and 1 teaspoon of honey, if desired. Drink up to 2 cups daily. Never gulp teas used as a treatment; drink warm in sips.

EPHEDRA TINCTURE

Add 1 cup of powdered ephedra to 1 quart of brandy or vodka. Place in a warm area or sunny window for two weeks. Strain and bottle. The dosage is 10 to 15 drops under the tongue every 15 minutes until the asthma is relieved. Or you can add 1 teaspoon of the tincture to 1 cup boiling water to use as a tea.

EPHEDRA CAPSULES

Mix together 1 tablespoon each of ephedra, violet leaves or flowers, yerba santa, and ginger. Place in #00 capsules. The dosage is 2 capsules every 4 to 5 hours.

Extra Caution: Use ephedra recipes under a physician's guidance and only to relieve congestion for acute asthmatic conditions.

WILD CHERRY BARK
Prunus serotina

OTHER NAMES: Black berry, wild black cherry, wild cherry, rum cherry.
PART USED: Young, thin bark. The inner bark of stems can be collected in autumn and dried.
SIGNATURE: The signature of wild cherry bark is its gummy exudation.

Wild cherry contains malic acid and hydrocyanic acid in small amounts. The properties are best extracted using water. It is often used to prepare cough syrups since it helps relieve congestion. Wild cherry is very helpful in removing phlegm from the chest and throat. It is an astringent and a sedative. It calms the respiratory system.

Caution: Large amounts of hydrocyanic acid, found in the wild cherry plant, especially the leaves, can be poisonous. Do not take more than the recommended amount; overdose may cause diarrhea and upset stomach. Toxicity may cause twitching, spasms, and difficulty breathing and speaking. Do not take the herb during pregnancy.

WILD CHERRY BARK INFUSION

Place 1 ounce of wild cherry bark, 2 tablespoons of licorice root, and 1 tablespoon of cloves in a stainless-steel pan. Pour 2 pints of boiling water over the mixture, and simmer 15 minutes. Strain, measure, and add an equal amount of honey or 6 tablespoons of glycerin as a preservative. The dosage is 1 to 2 teaspoons of the tincture to 1 cup of boiling water.

WILD CHERRY SYRUP

Take a handful of wild cherry bark and add it to 1 quart of water. Boil down to 1 pint. Strain, measure, and add an equal amount of sugar. Bring to a low boil for 5 minutes. Add 2 ounces of glycerin and bottle. The dosage is 3 to 4 tablespoons throughout the day as needed.

MULLEIN
Verbascum thapsus

OTHER NAMES: Great mullein, velvet dock, lungwort, candlewick plant, flannel leaf, mullein dock, clown's lungwort, Aaron's rod, ice leaf, Jacob's staff, Peter's staff, shepherd's staff, fluffweed, old man's flannel, white mullein, beggar's blanket.
PART USED: Leaves, flowers, and root.
SIGNATURE: The leaves have the texture of flannel. The woolly hairs suggest a tickling sensation in the throat and bronchial tubes.

Mullein appears to have some antibiotic properties. It also contains abundant potassium and calcium phosphate. These two organic salts are essential for the nervous system. It also contains choline, sulfur, magnesium, hesperidin, and PABA. The rich vitamin content includes vitamins B_2, B_5, B_{12}, and D.

The leaves have long been used as a "tobacco" for asthmatics. Mullein, like eyebright and foxglove, is in the coxcomb family, but great mullein is the only plant in that family used as an asthma treatment.

In Ireland the herb is considered specific for tuberculosis, asthma, colds, coughs, and pneumonia. It can be added to many other herbs as a treatment for asthma.

MULLEIN DECOCTION

A strong decoction can be made by adding 6 ounces of mullein leaves and flowers to 1 quart of water. Bring the herb mixture to a low boil, and boil gently for 15 minutes. Strain, press, and continue to boil until you have about 1½ pints of fluid left. Add 6 ounces of glycerin, bottle, and refrigerate.

The dosage for adults is 1 to 2 tablespoons daily. If used for children, add 6 ounces of honey and reduce the dose to 1 to 2 teaspoons daily.

MULLEIN ANTIASTHMATIC INFUSION

Prepare an infusion by adding 1 tablespoon of mullein leaves to 1 cup of boiling water. Cover and steep 15 minutes. Strain and add honey, if desired. This can be used three to four times daily.

HOREHOUND
Marrubium vulgare

OTHER NAMES: Marvel, white horehound, common horehound.
PART USED: Leaves and flowering top.
SIGNATURE: The leaves stick when pressed together. This suggests that it would cling to toxins and mucus to remove them from the body.

Horehound is found in the mint family, so it contains many of the same antioxidants. Using a warm infusion promotes perspiration and decreases the thickness of mucus in the bronchial tubes and lungs. It also increases fluidity of the mucus for easy expulsion. Horehound has been used for centuries worldwide in cough remedies. Horehound contains iron, potassium, B-complex vitamins, and vitamins A, C, and E.

HOREHOUND COUGH REMEDY

Mix 1 cup of horehound, 2 cups of white pine needles, and ½ cup of cherry bark. Cover with 1 quart of water and bring to a boil. Continue boiling until the liquid is reduced to half. Strain and add 1 pint honey. Pour into a bottle and store. This cough remedy can be taken by the tablespoon as needed for a cough.

HOREHOUND HONEY

Boil 1 ounce of horehound in 1 pint of honey for 10 minutes. Strain and bottle. Take by tablespoon as needed for cough.

PLEURISY ROOT
Asclepias tuberosa

OTHER NAMES: Swallow wort, tuber root, butterfly weed, wind root, chigger flower, Indian paintbrush.
PART USED: Dried root. *Do NOT use the fresh root.*
SIGNATURE: The name indicates the herb's use.

Pleurisy root, a member of the milkweed family, removes excess mucus built up from the lungs. Ascepin is the principal active ingredient. The dried root is used as an expectorant in tincture or infusion form. It can be prepared as a decoction to remove mucus and promote perspiration in treatment of the respiratory tract.

Pleurisy root is often added to cough syrups because of its expectorant properties. Boneset is often combined with pleurisy root, as are many other herbs used for chest congestion or asthma.

PLEURISY ROOT DECOCTION

Place 1 tablespoon of the root in 1½ pints of boiling water along with 1 teaspoon of ginger root. Boil slowly for 15 minutes. Remove from heat and steep, covered, until cool. The dosage is 1 cup twice daily. Tincture of peppermint may be added for flavor.

If the powdered root is available, you can add ½ teaspoon of the powder to 1 tablespoon of honey and ingest it that way. However, the liquid decoction is faster-acting.

ELECAMPANE
Inula helenium

OTHER NAMES: Elf dock, velvet dock, aunee.
PART USED: The root.
SIGNATURE: The large yellow flowers are the signature.

Elecampane, which acts as a stimulant, is often combined with yarrow or white willow in a decoction. The herb is a demulcent and an antibiotic. Elecampane contains inulin, helenin, and alantol. It is specific for combating tuberculosis bacillus; it is also very useful for other lung disorders and for bronchial distress.

LUNG CONGESTION TREATMENT

Pour 2 cups of honey in a pan and heat slowly. Add 2 tablespoons of powdered elecampane to the honey and continue simmering for 15 minutes. Strain and bottle. Take 1 tablespoon three to four times daily for lung congestion or coughing.

ELECAMPANE MIX

Mix 2 tablespoons each of elecampane and white willow with 2 cups of cold water. Allow the mixture to sit, covered, for 2 hours. Bring to a quick boil, and reduce heat to a simmer for 15 minutes. Remove from heat and steep for another 15 minutes, covered. Strain and add 1 cup of honey. Take 1 to 2 tablespoons every couple hours as needed.

ELECAMPANE LOZENGES

Place 2 cups of sugar and 2 cups of water in a stainless-steel pan. Lay enough of sliced, fresh elecampane root in the pan so that all the roots are covered. Bring to a quick boil until the roots are tender. Strain the elecampane slices and reserve the liquid. Roll the candied slices in powdered sugar or powdered slippery elm bark and place on wax paper.

The reserved liquid can be used as a cough syrup.

SKUNK CABBAGE
Symplocarpus foetidus

OTHER NAMES: Meadow cabbage, polecat weed, swamp cabbage, fetid hellebore, dracontium, skunkweed.
PART USED: Roots are gathered in the autumn or early spring and dried carefully.
SIGNATURE: Skunk cabbage grows in swampy areas. This indicates use in chest afflictions or so-called wet disorders.

Skunk cabbage has been used for centuries as an active diaphoretic and expectorant for chronic asthmatic conditions. It prevents involuntary muscular contractions.

SKUNK CABBAGE EXPECTORANT

Mix together 1 tablespoon of skunk cabbage, 1 tablespoon of skullcap, 2 tablespoons of crampbark, and $^1/_2$ teaspoon of cloves or cinnamon to 1 quart of warm brandy. Allow the mixture to steep 24 hours in a very warm area. Strain and rebottle. The dosage is 2 tablespoons three times daily.

Add 1 teaspoon of the tincture to 1 cup of boiling water or tea; use as an expectorant.

ELDER
Sambucus nigra

OTHER NAMES: Sweet elder, dwarf elder, American elder, European elderberry.
PART USED: Leaves, fruit, flowers, and root.
SIGNATURE: Elder grows in wet areas.

The leaves and flowers are used to promote secretion of fluids. The berries are a good source of iron, and many herbalists combine the juice from elderberries with the juice of blackberries. As an aid for asthma treatment, it is used mainly in the tincture form.

The berries are a source of vitamin C and can be prepared as a jam or jelly. Elder flowers and peppermint tea are specific for discharging mucus from the body.

ELDER–PEPPERMINT TEA

Mix 1 cup each of elder flowers and peppermint. Pour 1 cup of boiling water over 1 tablespoon of the mixture. Allow to steep 10 minutes, covered. Strain and drink hot. Honey may be used to sweeten the tea, if desired. Keep the patient warm and repeat every 30 minutes until a free perspiration begins.

LOBELIA
Lobelia inflata

OTHER NAMES: Indian tobacco, cardinal flower, red lobelia, pokeweed, wild tobacco, asthma weed, gagweed, emetic weed.
PART USED: Leaves and flowers.
SIGNATURE: The seed pod or capsule becomes swollen when it's ready to be harvested. The swollen capsules suggest use in swelling or types of inflammation.

Lobelia has become specific for treatment of asthma, although it is never used alone. If a little is used, the herb acts as a stimulant; in larger doses it becomes a relaxant. Lobelia is used as an antidote to any type of poison and removes obstructions from every part of the body. Lobelia is beneficial for the whole body. It is a great for removing hard and ropey phlegm.

Coltsfoot is often used in combination with lobelia, along with skullcap, peppermint, spearmint, valerian, blue cohosh, ginger, or another stimulant.

Lobelia contains selenium, sulfur, alkaloids, and isolobeline, cheliclonic acid, salts of lime, iron oxide, and potassium. It is a cough suppressant and a relaxant, which makes it helpful in treatment of asthma.

Caution: Lobelia should not be taken in large amounts or for a prolonged period. It has nicotinelike effects on the body. Taking more than 50 mg of dried lobelia can suppress breathing, depress blood pressure, and even lead to coma.

LOBELIA TINCTURE

Place lobelia in a pint jar and cover completely with brandy or vodka. Allow it to sit several weeks in a warm area or sunny window, shaking frequently or at least daily. The dosage is 1 teaspoon in a cup of peppermint or other tea. Sweeten with honey if desired. Take every two to three hours as needed.

LOBELIA INFUSION

Mix together 1 ounce of lobelia, $\frac{1}{2}$ ounce of skullcap, $\frac{1}{2}$ ounce of peppermint, and 1 tablespoon of ginger or cloves. Pour $1\frac{1}{2}$ pints of boiling water over the mixture and steep, covered, for 30 minutes. Strain and take 1 to 2 tablespoons every 30 minutes, as needed.

LOBELIA COUGH SYRUP

Mix together 2 tablespoons each of lobelia, mullein, pleurisy root, wild cherry bark, horehound, blue cohosh, and 3 tablespoons of ele-campane root.

Pour 2 pints of water over the mixture and bring to a slow boil. Simmer 15 minutes; then remove from heat and steep covered until cool. Strain and measure. Add an equal amount of honey. Add cherry flavoring, if desired for taste. Take by the tablespoon as needed for cough.

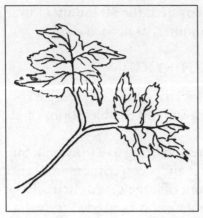

Goldenseal

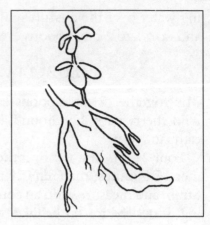

Licorice Root

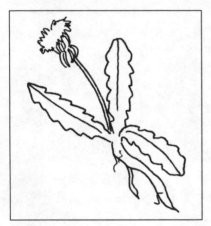

Dandelion

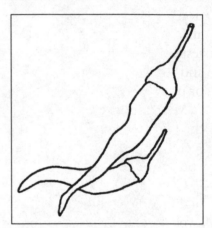

Cayenne Pepper

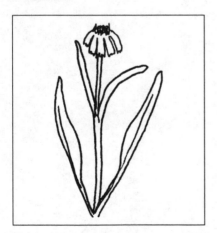

Echinacea

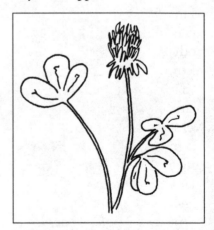

Red Clover

4. Chronic Fatigue Syndrome

Chronic fatigue syndrome (CFS) has all the symptoms of a viral infection. While you wait for the flulike symptoms to abate, you slowly realize something more is wrong. After many years, doctor visits, and tests, you recognize that chronic fatigue syndrome is a long-lasting and disabling disease. Researchers have still not determined the cause or process of the disease.

Many physicians even regard it as a psychiatric disorder, although the illness has been recognized worldwide. Some available treatments seem to help, but the bottom line is that you need to do as much as you can to help yourself lead a normal life again.

Current studies reveal that many CFS patients are highly intelligent, highly motivated people. They were the ones you turned to for the answer to any problem. Need volunteers? Mary never refuses. Need someone to care for your aging aunt? Ask Mary; she's there for you. Many of these people need to learn to set personal boundaries and to say no. Many CFS patients have found relief through integrating mind, body, spirit, and soul. Management requires multidisciplinary skills for recovery. Self-help as well as self-awareness are essential to healing.

The symptoms diagnosed often include depression or psychosomatic disorders. The patient may assume blame for this diagnosis and feel still more stress and guilt. Some physicians have had no label for the diagnosis. Jay Goldstein, M.D., director of the Chronic Fatigue Institute in Beverly Hills, California, says, "There is an increasing consensus that CFS is a virally induced cytokine-mediated psychoneuroimmunologic disorder that occurs in genetically predisposed individuals."

Although the disease is usually not life-threatening, it appears incurable and can do considerable damage to the immune system. It is estimated by the U.S. Centers for Disease Control in Atlanta, Georgia, that tens of thousands in the United States are infected with the disease. Often called the "yuppie disease," women are three times more likely to suffer from the virus. Many carriers are unaware that they have the virus because they have no symptoms.

Epstein-Barr virus, a member of the herpes family that causes shingles, chicken pox, and genital herpes, is the generally acknowledged cause of CFS. **Symptoms of chronic fatigue syndrome** include: (1) extreme fatigue, (2) recurrent upper respiratory infections, (3) anxiety, (4) depression, (5) mood swings, (6) memory loss, (7) inability to concentrate, (8) flulike symptoms, (9) swollen glands, (10) recurring sore throats, (11) sleep disturbances, and (12) fever.

We have growing evidence that antibiotics taken over a lifetime have an accumulative effect that could weaken the immune system and reduce resistance to illness. In our modern environment, we are exposed to many toxins, contaminants, and pollutants that can accumulate in the body.

Beginning to care for your own health needs first, in a self-disciplined way, sometimes causes trouble in relationships and families. Your family and friends should be informed about the nature of the disorder so that they can understand your frustration and heartbreak. Many patients respond well to relaxation therapy and learn to set personal boundaries. Stress reduction is important to your health; your friends and family need to be aware of your limitations.

VIRAL INFECTION REMEDY

1 tablespoon of licorice root
1 tablespoon of echinacea
1 tablespoon of goldenseal

Mix the licorice root, echinacea, and goldenseal and fill #00 capsules. Take 4 capsules four times daily for a week. Then quit for a week and begin again. This recipe increases the body's white-blood-cell count.

RECOMMENDED NUTRIENTS

There are different ways to build the body's immune system. Vitamin deficiencies can account for a lack of energy. A calcium supplement is important since it provides energy and has an important role in structuring RNA and DNA. Royal jelly can increase your energy level. Also important are vitamins B complex and C, selenium, zinc, kelp, and garlic. Kelp will supply your body with all the minerals it needs to help balance itself. Garlic acts as a wonderful natural antibiotic.

Vitamin B Complex   Take 100 mg three times daily.
Vitamin C   Take 3,000 to 8,000 mg daily.
Calcium   Take 1,500 mg daily.
Selenium   Take 100 mcg daily.
Zinc   Take 50 mg daily.
Kelp   Take 8 tablets daily.
Garlic   Take 2 capsules three times daily, with meals.
Royal Jelly   Take 2 capsules daily.

Your diet also plays an important part in regaining your health. Avoid a diet high in fat and sugar and low in fiber. Also avoid any processed foods. You should eat fresh fruits and vegetables that are organically grown. See chapter 10 for valuable food and herb sources of nutrients that you can add to your diet or take as teas.

HELPFUL HERBS

Herbal supplements can help you get the vitamins and minerals you need in your diet. There are many different ways to use herbs. Learn to prepare tinctures, teas, or capsules to regain your health. If the body is kept as clean as possible—free of toxins, drugs, and environmental poisons—your immune system will respond better. And the stronger the immune system, the faster your body will respond.

These herbs may be helpful for chronic fatigue syndrome: goldenseal, gotu kola, cayenne pepper, black cohosh, echinacea root, licorice root, Siberian ginseng, pau d'arco, dandelion, and red clover. Here are some herbs and herbal remedies to help you regain control of your health.

GOLDENSEAL
Hydrastis canadensis

OTHER NAMES: Ground raspberry, turmeric, orangeroot, yellow root, yellow puccoon.

PART USED: Root.

SIGNATURE: The yellow root and the red berries suggest use for the blood, liver, and urinary tract.

Goldenseal is an antibiotic and antiseptic used to help reduce infections. It contains alkaloids, berberine, and hydrastine, which has an effect on various infectious agents. It has been found to be effective against *Escherichia coli,* tuberculosis, streptococcus, and *Staphylococcus aureus* infections. Goldenseal is also an effective neural and glandular tonic. It can destroy bacteria in the gastrointestinal tract. Berberine is one of the few agents found to be effective against the water contamination of *Giardia*. Drinking water is becoming dangerous to our health.

Goldenseal also contains calcium, chlorine, choline, inositol, iron, potassium, manganese, phosphorus, and vitamins A, B complex, C, and E.

Usage of goldenseal should be alternated with acidophilus since it has a long-term effect upon the intestinal flora.

Caution: Avoid prolonged use. Since goldenseal is a potent herb, use it only under the direction of a physician or certified herbalist or nutritionist. Do not use goldenseal during pregnancy. Avoid it if you are allergic to ragweed.

GOLDENSEAL–JUNIPER BERRY REMEDY

This combination can be made into a tea, tincture, or capsule. To prepare the tea, place 1 teaspoon each of the goldenseal and juniper berries in a cup. Pour 1 cup of boiling water over the herb mixture and cover. Steep 10 minutes. Strain and drink. Drink several cups daily.

To prepare the tincture, place 1 tablespoon each of goldenseal and juniper berries in a pint jar. Pour 1 cup of vodka over the herbs and cap tightly. Place the jar in a warm area or sunny window and allow it to stand for several weeks. Strain and store in a sterile bottle. The dosage is 1 to 4 droppers added to any tea, juice, or water.

GOLDENSEAL CAPSULES

1 tablespoon of powdered goldenseal
1 tablespoon of powdered garlic
1 tablespoon of powdered juniper berries

Combine the goldenseal, garlic, and juniper berries. Mix well and fill #00 capsules. The dosage is 2 capsules three times daily with meals.

GINGER-GOLDENSEAL CAPSULES

> 1 tablespoon of goldenseal
> 1 teaspoon of ginger
> 1 tablespoon of licorice root
> 1 tablespoon of gotu kola

Combine goldenseal, ginger, licorice root, and gotu kola. Mix well and place into #2 capsules. Ginger is used as a catalyst, the licorice root feeds the adrenal glands, and the gotu kola helps combat fatigue. The suggested dosage is 2 capsules at least three times daily.

GOTU KOLA
Centella asiatica (umbelliferae)

PART USED: Leaves.

This is a tropically grown herb widely used in ayurvedic medicine. It has definite antifungal and antibacterial action. Its antibiotic properties are found in asiaticoside, one of many triterpene saponins. Asiaticoside is a cell proliferate. The volatile oils in the herb act as both a diuretic and blood purifier. Asians use it as a whole-body tonic.

Gotu kola contains potassium, sodium, iron, cobalt, calcium, manganese, magnesium, selenium, a trace of zinc, chromium, and vitamins A, B_1, B_3, C, and K. It also contains theobromine.

GLANDULAR TONIC

A combination of cayenne pepper (capsicum), ginseng, and gotu kola slowly increases energy physically and mentally. This mixture has been used for people recovering from a "nervous breakdown." Gotu kola helps build good adrenal health and stimulates the central nervous system.

> 1 tablespoon of ginseng
> 1 tablespoon of gotu kola
> 1 teaspoon of cayenne pepper (capsicum)

Mix ginseng, gotu kola, and cayenne pepper well and fill #00 capsules. The suggested dosage is 2 to 10 capsules daily.

IMMUNE-SYSTEM BUILDER

Echinacea is a well-known immune-system builder which helps fight off infections. This particular mixture stimulates the lymphatic system and increases the white-blood-cell count. Studies have found that echinacea's effects work only for about two weeks. After that the herb has no effect. One way to manage this effect is to take the herb for about two weeks, stop the treatment, then continue it two weeks later.

1 tablespoon of powdered echinacea
1 tablespoon of powdered gotu kola

Mix echinacea and gotu kola powders and fill #00 capsules. The suggested dosage is 2 to 6 capsules daily for two weeks. Stop and resume two weeks later.

RED CLOVER MIXTURE

2 tablespoons of powdered gotu kola
1 tablespoon of powdered Siberian ginseng
2 tablespoons of powdered red clover

Mix gotu kola, Siberian ginseng, and red clover, and fill #00 capsules. The suggested dosage is 2 to 6 capsules daily.

A tea or tincture can be made from any of the mixtures. If preparing a tea, add 1 to 2 teaspoons of the different herb mixtures to 1 cup of boiling water. Cover and steep 10 to 15 minutes. Strain and drink.

CAYENNE PEPPER
Capsicum annum

OTHER NAMES: Bird pepper, red pepper, African pepper.
PART USED: Fruit.
SIGNATURE: The red pod signifies blood cleansing.

Cayenne pepper, or capsicum, is often used with other herbs as a catalyst since it increases the absorption and effectiveness of almost any herbal formula. It aids circulation. Some people cannot take capsicum since it can cause stomach upset or an allergic (arthritislike) reaction, and it should NOT be taken as a long-term treatment.

It is a good source of folic acid, PABA, and vitamins A, C, B_1, B_2, B_3, B_6, and B_9. It is also a source of silicon, calcium, magnesium, iron, potassium, selenium, phosphorus, chromium, cobalt, and zinc. The chemicals it contains include capsacutin, capsaicin, capsico, capsanthine, and apsaicine.

Animal studies have demonstrated that capsicum given with ginseng and gotu kola provides resistance to stress. Stress can quickly deplete your immune system.

If preparing tinctures using cayenne pepper (capsicum), add the capsicum tincture to other teas or water about twice a week as a tonic for the immune system. Don't try to take the tincture under the tongue. Capsicum can cause burns or discomfort to this tender area.

Caution: Cayenne pepper (capsicum), a member of the nightshade family, contains solanine, which can irritate joints.

BLACK COHOSH
Cimicifuga racemosa

OTHER NAMES: Black snakeroot, rattletop, rattleroot, bugbane, bugwort, squaw root.
PART USED: Roots and rhizomes.
SIGNATURE: Twisted knotty root.

Black cohosh was one of the main ingredients of Lydia Pinkham's Vegetable Compound, used for menstrual discomfort. The herb is a hypotensive and a vasodilator; it lowers blood pressure. It has been used extensively as a tonic for the central nervous system. Black cohosh is also used as a muscle relaxant. It has sedative and antispasmodic properties if used fresh. Native Americans have long used it as an antidote for snake bites. It is also used as a heart tonic. Take only small doses since it can upset the stomach. The herb is antiinflammatory.

Black cohosh contains racemosin, triterpenes, actaeine, cimicifungin, palmitic acid, isoferulic acid, oleic acid, tannins, calcium, chromium, iron, phosphorus, chlorine, sodium, potassium, zinc, iodine, silicon, fluorine, pantothenic acid, and vitamins A and B complex.

Black cohosh is often used mixed with blessed thistle. The blessed thistle, also called holy thistle, is used to strengthen the whole immune system. The active ingredient in blessed thistle is niacin, somewhat like salicin, present in white willow. The herb is good for general aches and pains.

Caution: Do not use black cohosh if you are pregnant or have a chronic disease.

BLACK COHOSH TONIC

1 tablespoon of black cohosh
2 tablespoons of blessed thistle

Combine black cohosh and blessed thistle. If you are preparing it as a tincture, place the herbs in a pint jar and pour $1\frac{1}{2}$ cups of vodka over them. Cover and allow the jar to stand for two weeks. Strain and place the mixture in a sterile bottle. Take $\frac{1}{2}$ dropper in tea, water, or juice once or twice a day for several weeks. This tonic can also be taken directly under the tongue.

To prepare a tea, mix $\frac{1}{2}$ teaspoon of black cohosh and 1 teaspoon of blessed thistle in a cup. Pour 1 cup of boiling water over the herbs and cover. Steep 10 minutes and drink daily for a week, if desired.

WHOLE-BODY TONIC

Goldenseal is known for its tonic effect upon the body. Combining it with black cohosh makes an effective neural and glandular tonic. Goldenseal contains antibiotic properties.

Combine 1 tablespoon of goldenseal and 1 teaspoon of black cohosh. Mix and add 2 teaspoons of the dry mixture to 1 cup of boiling water. Steep 10 minutes, covered, and strain. Take 1 cup with every meal. The combined dry herbs can also be used in #00 capsules. The recommended dosage is 2 capsules three times daily.

BURDOCK–BLACK COHOSH TONIC

Burdock is a well-known blood cleanser. Combining it with black cohosh has an effect upon the whole immune system. Black cohosh has diuretic properties; so, blood impurities removed by the burdock will pass through the urinary tract. Adding ginger to the mix will hasten the process.

> 1 tablespoon of black cohosh
> 2 tablespoons of burdock
> $^1/_2$ teaspoon of ginger

Combine black cohosh, burdock, and ginger. This is best used as a tea. After mixing the herbs, place 1 teaspoon of the herb mixture in a cup. Add 1 cup of boiling water and cover. Steep 10 to 15 minutes. Drink several cups per day for one week. These mixed dry herbs can also be placed in #00 capsules. Take 2 capsules three times daily.

ECHINACEA
Echinacea purpurea

OTHER NAMES: Purple coneflower, black Samson, rudbeckia.
PART USED: Root and leaves.
SIGNATURE: The signature is the color of the flower and the conical head of florets.

Echinacea has antiviral, antiinflammatory, antifungal, and antibiotic properties. The herb is widely used for treating colds and flu for this reason. Studies suggest that echinacea can build up the immune system if used for 7 to 10 days. However, taking it longer than that really has no beneficial effect. After taking the herb for two weeks, stop, and do not resume use until two weeks later to get maximum results.

Echinacea is also used extensively as a tonic for the lymphatic system and to reduce swollen glands. Alcohol destroys the polysaccharides in echinacea, which stimulate the immune system, so it is best not to prepare tinctures using this herb.

The herb contains echinacen, echinacin B, betaine, echinacoside, echinolone, enzymes, inulin, inuloid, polyacetylene compounds, polysaccharides, arabinose, and fructose. Also present are calcium, cobalt, potassium, phosphorus, niacin, manganese, magnesium, sodium, zinc, copper, sulfur, iron, and vitamins A, C, and E.

ECHINACEA BLOOD PURIFIER

>1 tablespoon of burdock root
>1 tablespoon of red clover blossoms
>1 tablespoon of echinacea leaves
>2 tablespoons of apple pectin

Mix burdock root, red clover blossoms, echinacea leaves, and apple pectin. All these herbs have blood-cleansing properties. Place 2 teaspoons of the mixture in a cup. Pour 1 cup of boiling water over the herbs. Cover and steep 15 to 20 minutes. Add honey to sweeten. Drink several cups per day for several weeks.

ECHINACEA TONIC

>1 tablespoon of powdered echinacea root
>1 tablespoon of powdered goldenseal
>2 tablespoons of powdered licorice root

Combine the echinacea root, goldenseal, and licorice root. Since licorice root feeds the adrenal glands, it helps provide energy if taken long term. Mix the herbs well and fill #00 capsules. The suggested dosage is 2 to 8 capsules daily for two weeks. Stop and renew usage.

LICORICE ROOT
Glycyrrhiza glabra

OTHER NAMES: Sweet root, sweet wood.
PART USED: Dried root.
SIGNATURE: The signature is the long root and the sweet taste.

Licorice has properties similar in molecular structure to hormones from the adrenal cortex. It is helpful for relieving stress and promoting adrenal gland function. Licorice also has estrogenlike properties and can change the voice. Do not use if you have high blood pressure.

The Chinese use the root extensively as a tonic to give strength and endurance. The glycyrrhizin in licorice is antiinflammatory, and the flavonoids are responsible for its antibacterial and antifungal action. It is used to treat all blood disorders.

Licorice contains glycyrrhizin, inositol, asparagine, choline, fat, lecithin, pentacyclic terpenes, and the bioflavonoids licoflavonal, apigenin, liquiritin, and others. Minerals included are chromium, iron, magnesium, phosphorus, silicon, and sodium. It is also high in potassium and contains pantothenic acid, PABA, biotin, and vitamins B_1, B_2, B_3, B_6, and E.

Caution: Do not use licorice during pregnancy. Also avoid the herb if you have diabetes, heart disease, high blood pressure, a history of stroke, or glaucoma.

LICORICE TONIC

Use 2 to 4 tablespoons of the fresh licorice root or 1 teaspoon of the dried root per cup of boiling water. Make a tonic tincture by placing 2 tablespoons of the dried root in a pint jar. Add 2 cups of vodka and cover. Allow the mixture to sit at least two weeks before straining. Place the tincture directly under the tongue or add 1 to 2 droppers to tea water or juice.

LICORICE ENERGY CAPSULES

1 tablespoon of powdered dandelion root
1 tablespoon of powdered ginseng
2 tablespoons of powdered licorice root
1 tablespoon of powdered chickweed

Combine powdered dandelion root, ginseng, licorice root, and chickweed. Place powdered herbs in #00 capsules after mixing well. Take 2 capsules three times a day with meals.

LICORICE COMBINATION TONIC

1 tablespoon of dong quai
1 tablespoon of licorice root
1 tablespoon of ginseng
1 tablespoon of echinacea

Combine the herbs and use them in capsule form or drink them as a tea. Use 1 teaspoon in 1 cup of boiling water as a tea. If you use capsules, take 2 to 8 #00 capsules daily for two weeks.

SIBERIAN GINSENG
Eleuthrococcus senticosus

OTHER NAMES: Life everlasting, seed of earth, panacea, root of life, santa root.
PART USED: Roots and leaves.
SIGNATURE: The spiny shrub has a carrotlike root.

Siberian ginseng should not to be confused with Chinese or Korean ginseng (*Panax ginseng*). Siberian ginseng is a cousin of American ginseng (*Panax quinquifolium*), but native to Korea, China, and Siberia.

This ginseng is used primarily for immune deficiency, to improve memory, and to enhance endurance. Siberian ginseng contains triterpenoid saponins known as adaptogens. These saponins are not the same types found in panax ginseng. These nontoxic compounds increase resistance to emotional, chemical, and physical stress, and they can increase the activity of natural killer cells.

Siberian ginseng stimulates and strengthens adrenal and thyroid hormones. It is often used during cocaine withdrawal. The herb contains sodium, magnesium, iron, potassium, calcium, panaxosides, ginsenosides, arabinose, and vitamins A, B_3, B_{12}, C, and E.

Caution: Do not use Siberian ginseng if you have heart or circulatory disorders, high blood pressure, or hypoglycemia.

SIBERIAN GINSENG TONIC

Mix 2 ounces of honey with 1 ounce of Siberian ginseng. Add 40 drops of wintergreen oil. Mix well and add 1 teaspoon of this herbal mixture to 1 cup of hot water or tea. Drink as often as desired.

SIBERIAN GINSENG TEA

2 tablespoons of Siberian ginseng
2 tablespoons of saw palmetto

2 tablespoons of gotu kola
2 tablespoons of blessed thistle

Mix the herbs and place 1 to 2 teaspoons of them in 1 cup boiling water. Steep 10 minutes and strain. Add honey to sweeten, if desired.

GINSENG CAPSULES

1 tablespoon of Siberian ginseng
1 tablespoon of licorice root
1 tablespoon of black cohosh
1 tablespoon of gotu kola

Mix the herbs well and fill #00 capsules. The recommended dosage is 2 to 10 capsules daily for two weeks. Stop taking them after two weeks and go back on them for two weeks.

PAU D'ARCO
Tabebuia heptaphylla

OTHER NAMES: Taheebo, lapacho, ipe.
PART USED: Inner bark.
SIGNATURE: Although there are many species, the trees with the red, pink, or violet flowers are used medicinally. The color of the flowers suggests blood-cleansing properties.

Pau d'arco acts as an antibacterial and antifungal agent with healing effects. This good blood cleanser is known as a cancer remedy. The remedy consists of a tea brewed from the inner bark. This astringent and antibiotic is said to fight malaria, inhibit tumors, and cure leukemia.

It contains lapachol, naphthaquinones, and tannins, all thought to be antifungal. Pau d'arco also contains chrysophanic acid, fixed oils, resin, and sitosterol saponins, among others. Minerals present are calcium, cobalt, potassium, phosphorus, and magnesium, and vitamins present are A and C.

It can be used as a treatment for yeast infections by adding 1 teaspoon of the herb to 1 cup boiling water, taken three times daily.

PAU D'ARCO BLOOD CLEANSER TONIC

> 1 tablespoon of powdered yellow dock
> 1 tablespoon of powdered pau d'arco
> 1 tablespoon of powdered plantain leaves

Mix the powdered herbs and fill #00 capsules. The plantain acts as a diuretic that moves the toxins out through the urinary system. Take 2 capsules four times daily for two weeks.

PAU D'ARCO ANTIBIOTIC TREATMENT

> 1 tablespoon of powdered yarrow
> 1 tablespoon of powdered pau d'arco
> 1 tablespoon of powdered Siberian ginseng

Mix the herbs and fill #00 capsules. Take 2 capsules three times daily with meals for one to two weeks.

DANDELION
Taraxacum officinale

OTHER NAMES: Lion's tooth, cankerwort, wild endive, common dandelion, blow ball.
PART USED: All parts, but the root is favored medicinally.
SIGNATURE: The yellow flowers and the long tap root are the plant's signature.

Dandelion, a member of the sunflower family, affects the endocrine glands, and the circulatory and digestive systems. The wide distribution of the plant has been said to be Mother's Nature way of telling us that we all need to incorporate dandelion into our diet. The flowers are used to prepare jellies and wines. The leaves have long been used as a potherb or in salads, and the root has many well-known medicinal properties.

Dandelion is used extensively as a treatment for pancreatic, kidney, circulatory, and blood disorders. It helps balance the intestinal flora and helps absorb toxins from the intestines. The herb is bacteriostatic, fungistatic, and antispasmodic, and it can act as a diaphoretic.

Dandelion is one of the few herbs in which very small amounts of its properties are lost when drying the plant or root. The plant is high in minerals and contains calcium, iron, sodium, sulfur, potassium, phosphorus, magnesium, and a trace of zinc. It also contains biotin, folic acid, pantothenic acid, PABA, bioflavonoids, and is also high in beta-carotene and has vitamins A, B_1, B_2, B_3, B_6, B_{12}, C, and E.

Add the leaves to salads and other dishes as a dietary supplement.

DANDELION BLOOD CLEANSER

1 tablespoon of powdered chickweed
1 tablespoon of powdered licorice root
2 tablespoons of powdered dandelion root

Mix the herbs and fill #00 capsules. Take 2 to 10 capsules daily for several weeks.

DANDELION–JUNIPER BERRY TONIC

1 tablespoon of juniper berries
1 tablespoon of cut dandelion root

Add two teaspoons of the mixture of herbs to 1 cup of boiling water. Cover and steep 15 minutes. Drink several cups per day with meals.

RED CLOVER
Trifolium pratense

OTHER NAMES: Cleaver grass, cow grass, purple clover, trefoil.
PART USED: The head or flowers.
SIGNATURE: The color of the blossoms indicate use as a blood cleanser.

Red clover is used as a blood purifier, and because it is so high in nutritive value, it acts as a preventive as well as a remedy or treatment. This dependable nutritive supplement has been used to reduce tumors and lumps. It has antibiotic action against several bacteria, including the pathogen that causes tuberculosis. The herb also contains estrogenic and antispasmodic properties. Used with chaparral, red clover is considered a cancer remedy. Many also add dandelion to the Essiac cancer recipe as a preventive and treatment.

Red clover contains coumaric acid, coumestrol, saponins, salicylic acid, salicylate, biotin, and the minerals manganese, calcium, phosphorus, and sodium. It is high in potassium. Vitamins included are A, B_1, B_2, B_3 B_5, B_{12}, C, and bioflavonoids.

If using the fresh root, use 1 to 2 tablespoons of the herb to each cup of boiling water. The dried root can be reduced to 1 to 2 teaspoons for each cup.

RED CLOVER TINCTURE TONIC

> 1 tablespoon of red clover
> 1 tablespoon of dandelion root
> 1 tablespoon of pau d'arco
> 1 tablespoon of rose hips
> 1 tablespoon of licorice root

Mix the herbs and place them in a pint jar. Pour 2 cups of vodka over the herbs and cover tightly. Allow the mixture to sit for at least two weeks before straining. Take $1/2$ dropper under the tongue two times daily, or add 1 teaspoon of the tincture to 1 cup of tea or hot water. Honey can be added as a sweetener.

DANDELION CAPSULES

Powder dandelion roots and add them to #00 capsules. The dosage may be up to 10 capsules daily.

FIELD TONIC

> 1 tablespoon of dandelion root
> 1 tablespoon of chickweed
> 1 tablespoon of red clover blossoms
> 1 tablespoon of echinacea leaves

Mix herbs well and place 1 to 2 teaspoons in 1 cup of boiling water. Cover and steep 15 minutes. Strain and add honey. Drink several cups per day for several weeks.

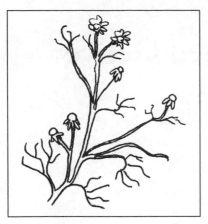

Chamomile

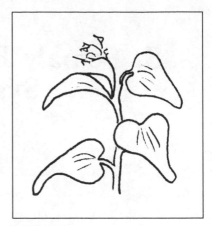

Wild Yam

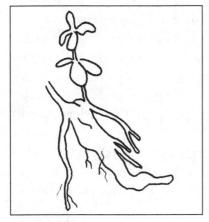

Licorice Root

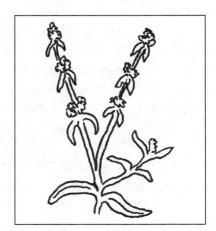

Pennyroyal

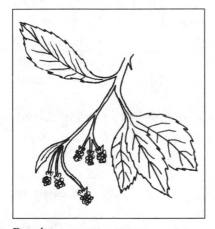

Raspberry

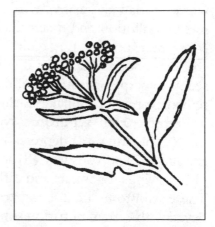

Elder

5. Female Reproductive System

Today women have many problems with their reproductive organs. And it appears that women are having these problems at a much younger age than in previous decades. This could be related to many different things, like nutrition, genetics, and environmental contaminants. Some studies suggest that the main problem is genetic, due to the presence of DDT, an insecticide found in virtually every waterway system in the civilized world. More women appear to have difficulty with the menstrual cycle, endometriosis, and related disorders than in the past.

Studies now reveal that low sperm count in the male population is usually the chief cause of infertility. However, this chapter deals with female disorders; we will discuss disorders of the male reproductive system in chapter 6.

Premenstrual syndrome (PMS) is a widespread problem for women today, and many herbal remedies can help. Here both environmental pollution and dietary habits appear to trigger the syndrome. Most meat, poultry, fish, grains, legumes, and produce in the Western world are not as healthy and wholesome as they once were. And this seems to perpetuate any genetic failings. For PMS, review both herbal remedies and nutritional guidelines.

Premenstrual syndrome symptoms include: (1) muscle cramping, (2) bloating, (3) depression, (4) headaches, (5) insomnia, (6) irritability, (7) nervousness, (8) acne, (9) tender breasts, (10) joint pain, (11) cravings for sweets and carbohydrates, and (12) water retention. These symptoms are not easy to live with. But PMS may be easily relieved with certain nutrition supplements.

The main reason women experience these symptoms is that the blood calcium in your body begins to drop about ten days before your period, and it continues to drop into the third day after your period begins. One solution is to increase your intake of calcium several days before your period begins. Just taking a calcium supplement, however, will not cover all your body's needs, so you want to include foods high in calcium in your diet. These foods are great to eat any time, but they are especially necessary to your body and should be added to your daily diet during the two-week time slot (ten or eleven days before, plus the first three days of, your period).

PMS symptoms are your body's way of telling you that you have an imbalance of prolactin and estrogen as well as thyroid and adrenal hormones. It is the liver's job to break down hormones and cleanse the body of toxins and metabolic wastes. But if the liver is over-loaded, the whole body becomes poisoned, and the liver becomes congested with estrogen components. Then the liver is unable to do its job. This creates premenstrual syndrome and other reproductive system disorders.

RECOMMENDED NUTRIENTS

In addition to calcium, vitamin B complex reduces premenstrual tension. Besides B vitamins, the liver needs protein to convert hormones released before menstruation into less powerful hormones. It may take several months before the B vitamins help you. Since brewer's yeast contains many B vitamins, you could begin taking it on a regular basis. Also, include a diet rich in protein to get maximum use of the B-complex vitamins. See chapter 10 for herbs and foods rich in B vitamins and in calcium.

HELPFUL HERBS FOR PREMENSTRUAL SYNDROME

Here are some recipes using herbs that will help relieve the symptoms of premenstrual syndrome. Also include herbs in your diet that are high in nutrients recommended for PMS. See chapter 10.

CORNSILK DIURETIC TEA

Take several tablespoons of cornsilk and place it in a cup. Pour 1 cup of boiling water over the herb, cover, and steep 10 to 15 minutes. Strain and drink.

PMS TEA

1 tablespoon of cramp bark
1 tablespoon of nettle leaves
1 tablespoon of strawberry leaves
1 tablespoon of peppermint leaves
1 tablespoon of black cohosh
1 tablespoon of wild yam root
2 tablespoons of gotu kola
5 tablespoons of dong quai

Mix the herbs. Take 5 tablespoons of the herb mixture and pour 1 quart of boiling water over it. Cover and steep 15 minutes. Drink slowly throughout the day. Sweeten with honey, if desired.

APPLE-PECTIN LIVER CLEANSER

Apple pectin is still the best cleanser I know. It can also act as a diuretic. Take as much in capsule form for three days as you can. I sometimes recommend up to 20 #00 capsules daily for three days to really clean the whole body. Follow this treatment with a potassium supplement, and choose several herbs high in B-complex vitamins.

NERVOUS SYSTEM TEA

1 tablespoon of violet leaves or flowers
1 tablespoon of white willow
1 tablespoon of dandelion
1 tablespoon of licorice root
3 tablespoons of hops
1 tablespoon of ginger

Mix violet, white willow, dandelion, licorice root, hops, and ginger. Take 1 teaspoon of the mixture and place it in a cup. Pour 1 cup of boiling water over the herbs. Cover and steep 10 to 15 minutes, strain, and drink warm. Sweeten with honey, if desired.

VALERIAN NERVE TREATMENT

Place valerian in capsules and take 2 capsules every four to five hours. Valerian calms nerves fast and its effects last about five hours. If you become drowsy, reduce the amount of the capsules. The herb is also a good sleep aid if you are having difficulty getting to sleep.

Menstrual cramps are common among women and girls. They are caused by prostaglandins, hormonelike substances that make the uterus contract. Good nutrition and some herbs will help reduce monthly distress due to painful cramps. If you have especially painful cramps, your body may need vitamin B_6, magnesium, and potassium in addition to calcium. If your cramps do not respond to a calcium supplement alone, add these nutrients to your diet. Calcium is not absorbed as well as the body's estrogen output lessens. A calcium deficiency can cause insomnia, depression, irritability, nervousness, and headaches. Both magnesium and vitamin D are needed for calcium absorption. Take 2 grams of calcium, 1,000 IU of vitamin D, and 1 gram of magnesium to quiet extremely painful cramps.

MENSTRUAL CRAMP REMEDY

A good mixture of herbs for cramps includes cramp bark, motherwort, white willow, and dong quai. Combine the herbs in equal parts and use 1 tablespoon to a cup of boiling water for a tea.

Excessive menstruation should be checked by your physician; this is one of the warning signs of cancer. But it could also be caused by an underactive thyroid, liver damage, or a vitamin E deficiency. Kelp tablets may help curb excessive menstrual flow. A thyroid condition may be partly relieved by adding protein, vitamin E, and iodine to your diet.

Amenorrhea, lack of a menstrual cycle, may be caused both by stress and nutritional deficiencies. Many women on low-calorie diets, or who are anorexic, miss their periods. A simple amenorrhea remedy, I'm told, is to apply a castor oil pack to the abdomen for up to one hour when one's period is late.

AMENORRHEA TEA

2 tablespoons of peppermint
3 tablespoons of pennyroyal
1 tablespoon of ginger or cinnamon bark

Simmer the ginger root or cinnamon bark on very low heat for 15 minutes in 1 pint of water. Remove from heat and add the pennyroyal and peppermint. Cover immediately and steep for 15 minutes. Strain and drink several cups daily.

Irregular flow or **cessation of menstrual flow** indicates general malnourishment or malabsorption of nutrients in the body. Vitamin E and B-complex vitamins are very helpful in correcting this condition.

Any adolescent just starting her monthly cycles may find that her periods are irregular. This may indicate a deficiency of zinc. Taking B_6 along with a zinc supplement helps establish regular cycles.

Endometriosis is a condition caused by endometrial cells that line the uterus leaving the uterus and beginning to grow elsewhere in the body. These stray cells have been found to be in or on the ovaries, fallopian tubes, bladder, intestines, behind the uterus, and in uterine musculature. Little is known about the cause of this disorder. It has been thought to be a major cause of infertility, and an estimated 10 to 15 percent of the female population suffer from it. Whatever the cause, this painful disorder is not easy to deal with. Most women who suffer from it have never been pregnant. One theory is that because these women have delayed childbearing, their reproductive organs gradually break down.

Endometriosis symptoms include: (1) intestinal discomfort, (2) bleeding between monthly cycles, (3) infertility, (4) excessive bleeding, (5) irregular periods, (6) pain during intercourse, (7) backache, (8) severe PMS symptoms, (9) passage of large clots, (10) nausea, (11) constipation, and (12) pain before, during, and after periods.

Taking 100 mg of vitamin B complex three times daily promotes hormone balance. Also, take 400 IU of vitamin E, slowly increasing the dosage to 1,000 IU. Vitamin B complex is particularly helpful in relieving nervous irritability. Take 2 tablets of kelp three times daily for essential minerals. If you take 100 mg of vitamin B_6 three times daily, it will help your water balance.

ENDOMETRIOSIS TEA

Mix together 1 tablespoon each of Siberian ginseng, raspberry leaves, and dong quai. Use 1 teaspoon per cup of boiling water. Cover and steep 10 minutes. Strain and add honey if desired. Drink at least once a day.

Dong quai is often used for problems associated with menopause, PMS, and hot flashes because it increases the effect of ovarian hormones.

PAU D'ARCO TINCTURE

Add 3 tablespoons of pau d'arco to a pint jar. Cover the herb with several inches of vodka or brandy. Screw on a tight lid, and place the jar in a sunny window for several weeks. Strain and bottle. Take 4 to 5 drops under the tongue three times daily for three weeks. Stop for one week and then resume for another three weeks, repeating the cycle as desired.

Menopause is often called change of life; it's the time in a woman's life when she stops ovulating. Usually symptoms last about 5 years. **Menopause symptoms** are: (1) shortness of breath, (2) depression, (3) heart palpitations, (4) hot flashes, and sometimes (4) a pronounced change in temperament.

Every woman begins this process at a different age, although you can expect it to begin between the ages of 45 and 55. In the post-menopausal phase, the production of estrogen in the body slows down. The endocrine glands assume the task of producing estrogen after the ovaries stop producing it. At this time, stress affects the adrenal glands, which often work overtime and produce smaller amounts of needed hormones. This may deepen depression, initially caused by the decrease of hormones in the body.

RECOMMENDED NUTRIENTS

Vitamin B complex taken with a calcium supplement (2,000 mg daily) is one of the best treatments for renewing the adrenal glands. This is a standard treatment for adrenal exhaustion. The recommended dosage is 100 mg of B-complex vitamins three times daily. Also helpful are kelp (3 tablets) and vitamin C (3,000 to 6,000 mg) taken daily to help control hot flashes.

HELPFUL HERBS

Besides these nutrients, some herbs may be helpful. Licorice root stimulates the production of estrogen. Also, an estrogen-production stimulant is Siberian ginseng. Ginseng also helps lessen the depression of menopause along with its other symptoms.

Caution: Do not take licorice if you have high blood pressure or cardiovascular disease. Also, do not use ginseng if you have hypoglycemia, high blood pressure, or a heart disorder.

MENOPAUSE SYMPTOM RELIEF

Mix 1 tablespoon each of black cohosh, raspberry leaves, gotu kola, dong quai, licorice root, and Siberian ginseng. Add 1 tablespoon of this herb mixture to a cup of boiling water for a tea.

Menopausal symptoms take time to regulate, so don't give up the treatment too fast. It may take several months before symptoms are reduced.

CALCIUM-RICH TEA

Mix 1 tablespoon each of any of the herbs in the chapter 10 list high in calcium. Add 1 teaspoon of the herb mixture to 1 cup of boiling water. Steep 10 to 15 minutes. Strain and drink two to three times daily. Good herbs for this tea are dandelion, licorice, juniper, clover, and eyebright.

HERBS WITH FEMALE HORMONES

Many herbs are good sources of female hormones: star grass, false unicorn, pussy willow, linden flowers, elder leaves and flowers, alfalfa, clover, sarsaparilla, pleurisy root, wild yam root, licorice root, wheat germ, garlic, and nettle.

These herbs can be taken alone or added to other remedies for menopause-related symptoms. The most widely used herb for female complaints is wild yam root. For centuries, women have favored this herb as a treatment because the body reacts to the diosgenin it contains much as it would to estrogen. Licorice also has estrogenlike properties and it helps nourish the adrenal glands, but licorice must not be used if you have high blood pressure or heart disease.

FEMALE HORMONE TEA

Try this easy remedy. Mix 1 tablespoon each of black cohosh (estrogenlike properties), licorice root (estrogenlike properties), valerian root (calms whole system), motherwort (strengthens nervous system), wild yam root (estrogenlike properties), skullcap (nervine; relieves headaches), and chamomile (mild relaxer).

Fill #00 capsules with this herb mixture. Take 2 capsules three times daily until symptoms abate. Thereafter, take 2 to 4 capsules daily.

HELPFUL HERBS

Here are more herbs you may find helpful for disorders of the female reproductive system: licorice root, black cohosh, wild yam root, pennyroyal, cramp bark, bearberry (uva ursi), false unicorn, goldenseal, raspberry, and ginseng.

LICORICE ROOT
Glycyrrhiza glabra

OTHER NAMES: Sweetwood, liquorice.
PART USED: Root.
SIGNATURE: The long root is slightly mucilaginous and sweet in taste.

Licorice root has recently been found to be a source of estrogenic hormones. It strengthens and modulates the activity of other herbs. It also adjusts blood salts and stimulates adrenal function. Licorice is high in pantothenic acid, biotin, manganese, PABA, phosphorus, protein, sugar, calcium, sodium, iodine, and vitamins E, B_2, and B_6.

It's important to add licorice to your herbal blends because it both stimulates the production of estrogens and promotes adrenal-gland function.

Caution: Do not use licorice if you have high blood pressure or cardiovascular disease.

FEMALE HORMONE TONIC

> 1 tablespoon of licorice root
> 1 tablespoon of gotu kola
> 1 tablespoon of dong quai,
> 1 tablespoon of black cohosh
> 1 tablespoon of raspberry leaves
> 1 tablespoon of Siberian ginseng

Mix the herbs well and place the mixture in #00 capsules. For menopausal symptoms, take 2 to 4 capsules daily.

WILD YAM ROOT
Dioscorea villosa

PART USED: Root.

Wild yam is used to treat dysmenorrhea, cramps, and menopausal symptoms. It is also used to prevent miscarriage. Wild yam contains compounds similar in structure to steroids. They must be digested, absorbed, and assimilated by the body before becoming hormones. Wild yam is now processed into pharmaceutical steroids and may be one of the most widely used herbs today in pharmaceutical production.

WILD YAM INFUSION

1 ounce of wild yam root
1 ounce of false unicorn
1 ounce of squaw vine
$1/2$ ounce of black haw
1 tablespoon of ginger

Mix and simmer the herbs in 1 quart of water for 20 minutes, covered. Strain. Take 1 small cup every three to four hours.

PENNYROYAL
Mentha pulegium or *Hedeoma pulegioides*

OTHER NAMES: Squaw mint, tickweed, mock pennyroyal, American pennyroyal, pudding grass.
PART USED: The top part of the herb.
SIGNATURE: Pennyroyal is aromatic, and it has properties similar to other herbs in the mint family.

Hot pennyroyal tea is used to treat suppressed menstruation. It contains the ketone puligone and volatile oils.

PENNYROYAL TEA

As a tea to bring your period, add 1 to 2 teaspoons of the herb to 1 cup boiling water. Cover and steep 15 minutes. Strain and drink hot.

CRAMP RELIEF TINCTURE

As a tincture treatment for cramps, mix together 1 tablespoon each of pennyroyal, cramp bark, ginger root, and valerian root. Put the herbs into a quart jar and fill the jar about two-thirds full with vodka or brandy. Put on a lid and place the jar in a sunny window. Allow it to stand for about two weeks. You can carry the treatment with you if it's in a tincture form. The dosage is 4 to 8 drops under the tongue.

Caution: Do NOT use pennyroyal during pregnancy.

CRAMP BARK
Viburnum opulus or *Viburnum prunifolium*

OTHER NAMES: True cramp bark, high bush, cranberry bush, sloe, black haw, arrowwood.
PART USED: Dried bark of stem or root.
SIGNATURE: Cramp bark grows in damp areas or along streams.

Cramp bark has long been recognized as a uterine sedative and tonic. It was used by Native Americans to treat both dysmenorrhea and discomfort during pregnancy. It prevents miscarriage caused by nervous disorders. Cramp bark contains phosphates of magnesium, calcium, and potassium.

TO REGULATE MENSTRUATION

Add 2 ounces of cramp bark to 1 quart of water. Boil gently for 20 minutes, covered. Strain and continue boiling until reduced to $3/4$ pint. Add 4 ounces of glycerin and cool. Bottle in a sterile container. The recommended dose is 1 to 3 tablespoons daily as needed to regulate menstruation.

CRAMP REMEDY

1 ounce of cramp bark
1 ounce of blue vervain

1 ounce of skullcap
1 ounce of wild yam
4 to 6 sticks of cinnamon bark

Place the herbs in 2 quarts of cold water. Allow the herb mixture to stand overnight. The next morning, bring it to a boil, lower the heat, and simmer gently for 30 minutes, covered. Strain and continue cooking until the liquid is reduced to 1 pint. Add 4 tablespoons of glycerin. Take 1 to 3 teaspoons in 1 cup of warm water.

CRAMP REMEDY WITH WINE

Warm 1 quart of wine. Add 1 ounce of cramp bark, $\frac{1}{2}$ ounce each of skunk cabbage and skullcap, and 1 teaspoon each of cinnamon and clove to the warm wine. Cap and allow the mixture to sit in a warm area or sunny window for at least 24 hours. Strain and rebottle. Take 1 to 2 tablespoons in 1 cup of hot water every two to three hours as needed for cramps.

BEARBERRY
Arctostaphylos uva-ursi

OTHER NAMES: Uva ursi, mountain box, upland cranberry, mealberry, rockberry, sandberry, bear's grape, creashak.
PART USED: Fruit and dried evergreen leaves.
SIGNATURE: A thick mass grows on rocky, sandy, and gravely areas, and the plant's red berries are its signature.

Do not use bearberry during pregnancy. Bearberry (uva ursi) contains potassium, arbutin, tannins, chlorine, ellagic acid, malic acid, and volatile oils. Uva ursi is a bitter and strong astringent. It is best taken with a mucilaginous diuretic herb like marshmallow. The herb can decrease menstrual flow.

FOR REDUCING MENSTRUAL FLOW

1 tablespoon of powdered uva ursi
1 tablespoon of powdered cranesbill root
1 tablespoon of powdered witch hazel leaves

1 tablespoon of powdered raspberry leaves
1 tablespoon of powdered papaya leaves
1 tablespoon of powdered shepherd's purse
1 tablespoon of powdered cramp bark

Mix the herbs and place them in #00 capsules. The recommended dose is 4 to 6 capsules daily. To prepare as a tea, place 1 teaspoon of the herb mixture into 1 cup of boiling water. Steep 10 minutes and strain. Drink 4 cups per day.

Cranesbill treats **menorrhagia,** abnormally heavy bleeding. Witch hazel has astringent properties. Raspberry leaves relax the smooth muscles of the uterus if they are in tone and contracts them if they're not toned.

Papaya leaves contain antihemolytic properties and also act as an emmenagogue. The herb promotes menstruation for young women who have delayed starting their periods, and it treats painful menstruation.

Black haw contains several uterine muscle relaxants. It also relieves painful menses and tones the reproductive system. Shepherd's purse is effective in treating menorrhagia. The properties in shepherd's purse coagulate blood. It tones the uterus and contains uterine-contracting properties.

FALSE UNICORN
Chamaelirium luteum

OTHER NAMES: Blazing-star, helonias, fairy-wand, rattlesnake, devil's bit.
PART USED: Root system.
SIGNATURE: False unicorn grows in moist, low areas. It has a yellowish color, so this indicates astringent properties.

The herb is as a uterine tonic in treating dysmenorrhea and amenorrhea. False unicorn is also used as a treatment for hot flashes.

HOT-FLASH TREATMENT

1 tablespoon of false unicorn
1 tablespoon of ginseng

1 tablespoon of licorice root
1 tablespoon of black cohosh
1 tablespoon of wild yam
1 tablespoon of blue vervain

Place the herbs in a quart jar and cover them using twice the amount of vodka or brandy as you have herbs. Place the covered jar in a sunny window or warm area for two weeks. Strain and bottle. Take 1 teaspoon of the tincture in 1 cup of tea or boiling water.

TEA FOR REDUCING MENSTRUAL FLOW

1 tablespoon of false unicorn root
1 tablespoon of raspberry leaves
1 tablespoon of cramp bark
1 tablespoon of bearberry (uva ursi) berries
1 tablespoon of ginger root
1 tablespoon of squaw vine

Mix the herbs and add 1 teaspoon of this mixture to 1 cup of boiling water. Cover and steep 15 minutes. Strain and drink warm. Drink 1 cup every hour or so, as needed.

FEMALE REPRODUCTIVE SYSTEM TONIC

1 tablespoon of dong quai
1 tablespoon of black cohosh
1 tablespoon of ginger root
1 tablespoon of raspberry leaves
1 tablespoon of marshmallow
1 tablespoon of cranesbill

Place the herbs in a quart jar and cover them with vodka or brandy— up to twice the amount of the herbs in the jar. Place the jar in a sunny window or warm area for about two weeks. Strain and bottle. Take the tincture directly under the tongue, or add 1 to 2 teaspoons of the tincture to 1 cup of hot tea or boiling water. Drink several cups per day, if desired.

RASPBERRY
Rubus idaeus

OTHER NAMES: Red raspberry, European raspberry, framboise.
PART USED: Leaves, root, and fruit.
SIGNATURE: The signature is the red fruit, sharp thorns, and taste of the root.

Native Americans used raspberry extensively during pregnancy to facilitate delivery. Raspberry relaxes the uterine muscles, regulates the hormones during pregnancy and delivery, and reduces cramps during menstruation. It can also decrease menstrual bleeding.

The herb contains pectin, silicon, citric acid, and vitamins C and D.

Use this recipe for menstrual disorders, morning sickness, hot flashes, or preparation for childbirth. Take a B-complex vitamin supplement with the tea or tincture. This recipe is especially helpful during the third trimester of pregnancy. It tones the uterus, relieves pain and discomfort, and helps relieve muscle spasms.

RASPBERRY TONIC

2 tablespoons of raspberry
1 tablespoon of black cohosh
1 tablespoon of dong quai
1 tablespoon of butcher's broom
1 tablespoon of squaw vine

Prepare the mixed herbs as a tincture with vodka or brandy, or add 1 to 2 teaspoons of the herb mixture to 1 cup of boiling water. Cover and steep 10 to 15 minutes. Strain and drink several cups per day. You can add the tincture to hot tea or water, or take it directly under the tongue.

GINSENG
Panax quinquefolius

OTHER NAMES: Man's health, five-finger, sang, ninsin, panax, pannag, red berry, American ginseng.

PART USED: Root.
SIGNATURE: The root resembles the human form.

Ginseng encourages natural estrogen production, decreases fatigue, and strengthens the adrenal glands.

It contains calcium, camphor, iron, saponin, gineosides, magnesium, manganese, potassium, and vitamins A and B_{12}. Ginseng directly stimulates the adrenocortical system and balances the female reproductive system.

GINSENG TONIC

2 tablespoons of ginseng
1 tablespoon of bearberry (uva ursi)
1 tablespoon of cramp bark
1 tablespoon of raspberry
1 tablespoon of black cohosh
1 tablespoon of wild yam

Mix the herbs well and fill #00 capsules. Use 2 capsules daily as a tonic. You can prepare this tonic as a tea, if desired. Use 1 to 2 teaspoons of the mixed herbs to 1 cup of boiling water. Cover and steep 10 to 15 minutes. Strain and drink 1 cup daily.

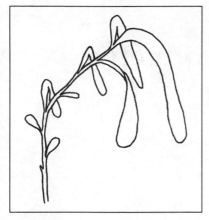

Horsetail

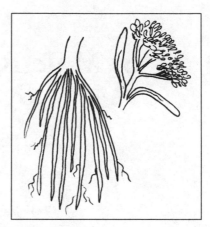

Joe-Pye Weed

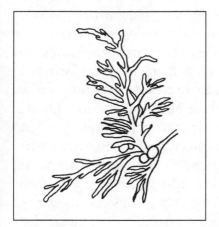

Juniper Berry

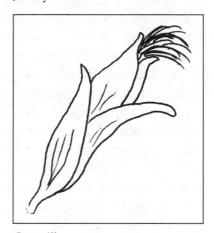

Cornsilk

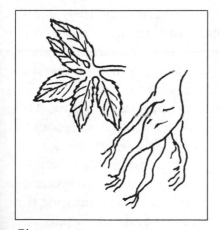

Ginseng

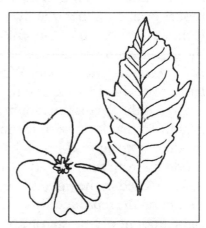

Marshmallow

6. Male Reproductive System

The health of the male reproductive system is important for many reasons, but sexual performance and infertility are usually what most concerns men.

Impotence can be expected now and then. All men experience it some time in their lives. Fatigue, too much alcohol, drug use, pressure in professional or personal life, and depression can cause temporary impotence. Physical and psychological factors also contribute to failure in achieving or maintaining an erection long enough to permit penetration.

Sex starts with the brain. Failure to achieve arousal, no matter what the stimulus, is a key to understanding impotence. Certain hormonal changes must occur. The male hormone testosterone must be in plentiful supply, circulating throughout the system. While men generate both testosterone and estrogen, testosterone must be generated in much greater amounts. The liver is responsible for maintaining hormonal balance. When the liver is damaged, whether by toxic effects from alcohol or other causes, liver function is impaired. This allows the female hormone estrogen to accumulate, which in turn neutralizes the effects of testosterone. When this happens, the breasts may enlarge, testes may shrink, and the sex drive may be reduced.

Even if the liver is functioning properly, the pituitary gland must be healthy so that it can secrete the hormone that stimulates the testes to produce testosterone. But if the testes are diseased, then no amount of prodding from the pituitary gland will force them to produce the hormone needed in the right amount to prepare the penis for an erection. Assuming the reproductive system is in good health and producing the right amount of testosterone, it is still possible that the nerve pathway is not intact or healthy. Many disorders, such as spinal injury, diabetes, or alcoholism can cause enough damage to prevent the brain-to-penis signal. Arteriosclerosis may also cause difficulty simply because it can affect the blood flow to the penis. The penis can become erect only when flooded with blood.

The number-one cause of impotence is an unresponsive emotional state. This can be caused by fatigue, boredom, anxiety, depression, sadness, or a deep emotional problem. When trying to determine the cause of impotence, review with your physician the medications you are currently taking. There are at least eighty different commonly prescribed drugs that may be responsible. Any mood-altering prescription drug is usually high on the list, along with drugs used to treat high blood pressure or heart disease. Brain tumors, Parkinson's disease, strokes, diabetes, and alcoholism can also cause impotence.

Premature ejaculation is most often caused by emotional problems. If a change in partners or masturbation works for you, then the most likely cause is emotional.

Infertility was once more common in females than males. Today many more males are infertile than females. Because soil worldwide is deficient in zinc, we can expect more male fertility problems. The sperm and prostate seminal fluid hold more zinc than any other cells in the human body. Studies in Iran and Egypt on young males who had undersized or immature genitalia have shown that when these young males were put on a diet high in zinc and iron, they grew rapidly and matured sexually. Zinc supplements promote sexual maturation.

RECOMMENDED NUTRIENTS FOR THE PROSTATE

Prostate problems can also be related to a zinc deficiency. Studies at St. James Hospital in Leeds, England, demonstrate that serum zinc is significantly lower in patients with prostate cancer. They also have a shortage of vitamin A. Deterioration of prostate tissue can be reversed by a vitamin A supplement in mice. Enlargement of the prostate also calls for copper, iron, manganese, and calcium supplements.

Sexual indifference indicates deficiencies of iron, copper, sulfur, manganese, phosphorus, and nitrogen. See chapter 10 for herbs and food high in these essential minerals.

For men, the most common disorder in the genitourinary system is in the prostate. Prostatitis, hypertrophy, and cancer are three of the most common disorders.

Prostatitis, however, is common in males of all ages. Usually, an infection from somewhere else in the body invades the prostate. Prostatitis can cause a blockage in the flow of urine from the bladder. The symptoms of acute prostatitis include pain between the scrotum and rectum, a burning sensation during urination, fever, and frequent urination, especially at night. Blood or pus may be present. Lower back pain and impotence may accompany chronic prostatitis. As the infection progresses, urination becomes more difficult.

For men over 50 years old, prostate enlargement or hypertrophy is common. When enlargement occurs, the gland presses on the urethral canal. This can cause retention of urine in the bladder, which can back up into the kidneys. This may cause extensive kidney damage. Symptoms of enlargement include frequent urination, especially at night, burning and pain on urination, and difficulty starting and stopping the flow.

Premature ejaculation, being unable to achieve or maintain an erection, and failing to ejaculate mean that sperm cannot impregnate the female ovum. Take a good vitamin supplement if you've checked out other medical possibilities and still have a problem with fertility. These vitamins may increase male fertility.

RECOMMENDED NUTRIENTS FOR MALE VITALITY

Vitamin A   Begin with 200 IU and increase slowly to between 400 and 1,000 IU daily.

Vitamin B Complex   Maintains a healthy nervous system.

Zinc   Take 80 mg of zinc daily, since this mineral is important for prostate function.

Vitamin C   This vitamin keeps sperm active and prevents it from clumping. Take 3,000 to 6,000 mg daily.

Vitamin B_6   This vitamin helps synthesize RNA and DNA, which contain genetic instruction for cell reproduction.

See chapter 10 for food and herbal sources of these important nutrients.

Prostate cancer is the third most common malignancy for men. Men under age 60 rarely get prostate cancer. Symptoms are often overlooked. Ninety percent of cases remain undetected until the disease is more difficult to treat. **Prostate cancer symptoms** are similar to hypertrophy: (1) blood in the urine, (2) frequent urination, and (3) a burning sensation during urination. Other warning signs include (4) repeated prostate infections and (5) a history of venereal diseases.

Of all the minerals needed for prostate health, zinc is most important. If you suffer from prostatitis, take 80 mg daily. To prevent the disorder, take 15 mg of zinc with 3 to 6 capsules of polyunsaturated fatty acids daily. Cold-pressed oils like sesame, olive, or safflower oil should be included in your daily diet. Also include brewer's yeast daily along with fruit, fruit juices, raw vegetables, seeds, nuts, dried beans, brown rice, and peas. One ounce daily of raw pumpkin seeds is a good preventive; these seeds are extremely high in zinc. Corn germ is extremely high in zinc and should be added to your daily diet.

Men who have had a vasectomy are three times more likely to develop prostate cancer. Many herbs can help prevent or treat prostate problems.

PROSTATITIS TREATMENT

$\frac{1}{2}$ cup of sea holly
$\frac{1}{2}$ cup of hydrangea root
$\frac{1}{2}$ cup of Joe-Pye weed
$\frac{1}{2}$ cup of marshmallow leaves or slippery elm

Place the herbs in a stainless-steel pan and pour 2 quarts of water over them. Bring to a boil and quickly reduce heat to simmer. Then simmer, covered, until the liquid is reduced to almost half. Cool, strain, and place in a sterile bottle. Take 3 to 4 tablespoons of the liquid three times daily. The decoction can be added to other teas, juice, or water.

If symptoms recur, see your physician. If blood is present in the urine, try the horsetail remedy.

HORSETAIL REMEDY

Mix equal parts of horsetail herb and hydrangea root. Cover completely with water and simmer until the liquid is reduced almost to half. Cool, strain, and bottle. Take 1 to 2 tablespoons of the remedy in 1 cup of hot water, or add it to other teas, juice, or coffee.

These herbs are helpful for the male reproductive system. They may be used alone or combined: juniper berries, saw palmetto, dong quai, cornsilk, hydrangea root, gotu kola leaves, couch grass, Siberian ginseng, and damiana.

JUNIPER BERRIES
Juniperus communis

OTHER NAMES: Juniper bush, common juniper.
PART USED: Berries.

Juniper berries have long been used to treat infections and help heal chronic urinary-tract infections. They are also very useful in treating prostatic hypertrophy. Juniper berries are also great for eliminating blood impurities.

The herb is considered a disinfectant and antiseptic. The berries contain vitamins A and C as well as the minerals zinc, selenium, potassium, chromium, calcium, iron, manganese, magnesium, phosphorus, and niacin.

PROSTATE HYPERTROPHY TREATMENT

Mix 3 tablespoons each of gotu kola and dried juniper berries. Put 2 teaspoons of the herb mixture in 1 cup of hot water. Cover and steep 15 minutes. Strain and drink several cups daily.

JUNIPER BERRY TINCTURE

To make a tincture, add 3 tablespoons of the berries to a pint jar. Fill the container with $1\frac{1}{2}$ cups of alcohol; vodka or brandy can be used. Place the jar in a sunny window for about two weeks, shaking occasionally. Strain and place in a sterile jar. Add up to 1 full dropper to tea, juice, or water. You can take several drops directly under the tongue several times a day instead of adding the tincture to another liquid.

Here's another good tincture. Add equal parts of goldenseal, juniper berries, gotu kola, and bearberry (urva ursi) to 1 quart of alcohol. Follow the procedure above. The dosage is the same.

SAW PALMETTO
Serenoa repens (Serenoa serrulata)

OTHER NAMES: Dwarf palmetto, sabal, fan palm, scrub palmetto.
PART USED: Berries.

Saw palmetto is used to reverse atrophy of the testes and other disorders of the male reproductive system. The berries reduce pain and swelling of an enlarged prostate due to an inflammation or infection. They also help the bladder empty because saw palmetto helps the bladder muscles contract. The herb is a mild aphrodisiac.

Saw palmetto is used extensively as a preventive. It contains selenium, iron, chromium, calcium, magnesium, manganese, phosphorus, potassium, zinc, silicon, and vitamins A and C.

Recent tests have shown that the berries have the ability to reduce prostate enlargement, due to an unidentified compound in the berries.

SAW PALMETTO REMEDY

For an enlarged prostate, fill #00 capsules with dried saw palmetto berries made into a powder. Take 3 to 6 capsules daily.

For treatment of an inflamed prostate, take 4 to 8 capsules daily. If you prefer a tea, add 1 to 3 teaspoons of the dried saw palmetto berries to 1 cup of boiling water. Cover and steep 15 minutes. Strain and drink at least twice daily.

PROSTATE AID

> 2 tablespoons of powdered saw palmetto berries
> 1 tablespoon of powdered parsley
> 1 tablespoon of powdered buchu leaves
> 1 tablespoon of cayenne pepper
> 2 tablespoons of kelp
> 2 tablespoons of powdered slippery elm

Mix the herbs well and fill #00 capsules. Take 2 capsules three times daily.

Use this mixture as a preventive or as a treatment for prostate problems. For herbs not already made into a powder, use a small, clean electric coffee grinder to reduce the herb to a powder. The cost is small and the results are great.

SAW PALMETTO–SIBERIAN GINSENG PROSTATE TEA

Mix equal parts of saw palmetto berries and Siberian ginseng. Add 1 to 3 teaspoons of the herb mixture to 1 cup of boiling water, cover, and steep 15 minutes. Strain and drink several times daily. This mixture can also be made into a tincture. Add 1 tablespoon of each of the herbs to 1 pint of alcohol and allow it to sit for several weeks. Tinctures are practical because you can place them in a small bottle to carry with you to work. Add the tincture to tea or another liquid several times daily or take it directly under the tongue. You can also purchase empty tea bags to fill with 1 to 3 tablespoons of the herb mixture. This is also an easy way to use the herbs at work. All you would need is hot water to make the tea, and you can discard the bag easily. This is helpful for prostate complaints.

DONG QUAI ROOT
Angelica sinensis

OTHER NAMES: Angelica.
PART USED: Root.

Dong quai increases the effect of testicular hormones. Black cohosh seems to help dong quai work more efficiently.

Tests have shown that dong quai protects the liver from the effects of harmful chemicals, and it increases the oxygen consumption of the liver. Chinese medicine considers it an aphrodisiac. Dong quai contains iron, selenium, silicon, chromium, calcium, magnesium, manganese, phosphorus, potassium, a trace of zinc, and vitamins A, B_{12}, and C.

DONG QUAI MIXTURE

1 tablespoon of slippery elm
2 tablespoons of dong quai
1 tablespoon of licorice root
1 tablespoon of black cohosh
1 tablespoon of ginger root

Mix the powdered herbs thoroughly and fill #00 capsules. Take 2 capsules three times daily.

Or make a tincture with vodka or brandy. Place the herbs in a quart jar and fill the jar with alcohol. Place the jar in a sunny window for two weeks. Strain and bottle in a sterile container. The tincture dosage is $^1/_2$ dropper directly under the tongue three times daily.

DONG QUAI TEA

> 1 tablespoon of dong quai
> 1 tablespoon of marshmallow root
> 1 tablespoon of juniper berries
> 1 tablespoon of licorice root
> 1 tablespoon of Siberian ginseng
> 1 tablespoon of ginger root

Place 1 to 2 teaspoons of the herb mixture in 1 cup of boiling water. Cover and steep for 10 to 15 minutes. Drink a cup of dong quai tea two times daily.

CORNSILK

PART USED: Silk from sweet corn.
SIGNATURE: The color of the silk suggests use for urinary problems.

Cornsilk is excellent for an enlarged prostate, kidney disorders, bladder infections, or any urinary dysfunction. It is especially useful for painful urination associated with the prostate gland. It also can be used as a treatment for hypertension, edema, and bedwetting.

Cornsilk has many useful minerals and vitamin K. It contains alkaloids, oxalic acid, ascorbic acid, malic acid, palmitic acid, pantothenic acid, silicon, and tartaric acid.

The only way to receive cornsilk's benefits is to prepare it as a tea.

MEN'S CORNSILK TEA

Take several tablespoons of the silk and place in a cup. Pour 1 cup of boiling water over the silk and cover. Steep 10 to 15 minutes. Drink several cups daily for up to three to four days. Stop, and then continue the following week for several days, if desired. Since cornsilk is a strong diuretic, it should not be used for long periods. It won't be necessary to use it longer than a few days since it seems to clear up the problem quickly.

If you are treating the kidneys, add 1 teaspoon of comfrey root to the cornsilk tea, since comfrey acts as a blood cleanser and kidney treatment.

Dry and save your own cornsilk for later use. This way you can ensure the purity of the silk and prepare as much as you like. When you shuck fresh corn to eat, just save the silk. Lay it on cheesecloth and place in an area that will get some air. Turn it at least once a day until it's dry. Store the dried silk in a tightly closed container.

HYDRANGEA ROOT
Hydrangea arborescens

OTHER NAMES: Sevenbarks, stone root, gravel root, hills-of-snow, wild hydrangea.
PART USED: Root.

Hydrangea contains iron, magnesium, manganese, calcium, potassium, selenium, zinc, chromium, and vitamins A, B_3, and C. It also contains several flavonoids, quercetin, and rutin that help reduce inflammation of the prostate. It is diuretic in nature and inhibits the formation of tumors. The root increases the production of urine and enhances the elimination capability of the urinary system. It is used to treat benign prostatic hypertrophy.

Caution: Do not consume hydrangea leaves, which contain cyanide. They are toxic.

HYDRANGEA TEA

To prepare a tea, add $1\frac{1}{2}$ teaspoons of dried hydrangea root to 1 cup of boiling water. Cover and steep 10 to 15 minutes. Strain and drink several cups daily.

HYDRANGEA TINCTURE

Place 4 tablespoons of the hydrangea root, chopped fine, into a pint jar. Add 2 cups of vodka or brandy to the jar and close tightly. Place the jar in the sun for two weeks, shaking daily. Strain and place the contents in a sterile container. Use 1 full dropper in 1 cup of hot water.

Drink several times daily. The tincture can also be placed directly under the tongue.

HYDRANGEA SYRUP

Place 1 cup of chopped hydrangea root in a stainless-steel pan. Pour 1 quart of water over the root. Bring to a fast boil, reduce heat, and simmer until the liquid is reduced to half. Strain and measure. Add an equal amount of sugar and bring the mixture to a rapid boil for about 10 minutes or until a syrup forms. Place the syrup in a sterile container. Refrigerate if desired; it will thicken. Or store it in a cool, dark place. The recommended dosage is several teaspoons daily.

GOTU KOLA
Centella asiatica (umbelleferae)

PART USED: Leaves.

Gotu kola is an antibiotic, bactericide, fungicide, and insecticide. It is also a blood purifier and a diuretic. It can help reduce inflammation of the genitourinary system.

An active constituent of gotu kola is asiaticoside, one of the triterpene saponins, which speeds healing by stimulating cell division. Cholesteremic steroids like beta-sitosterol help lower serum cholesterol levels.

Gotu kola has the minerals calcium, chromium, cobalt, iron, magnesium, manganese, phosphorus, potassium, selenium, silicon, sodium, zinc, and tin, and vitamins A, B_1, B_2, B_3, and C. It is used because it promotes prostate health. The herb can be taken as a tea, in capsules, or as a tincture.

GOTU KOLA TREATMENT

2 tablespoons of powdered gotu kola
2 tablespoons of powdered Siberian ginseng
1 tablespoon of powdered saw palmetto
1 tablespoon of powdered black cohosh

Mix the herbs thoroughly and fill #00 capsules. Take 2 capsules three times a day.

GOTU KOLA TINCTURE

Place ⅓ cup of gotu kola leaves in a pint jar. Cover the herb with 2 cups of vodka or brandy. Cover tightly and place in a sunny window for 2 to 4 weeks. Strain and add 1 teaspoon to 1 cup of hot water as a tea. Drink several cups daily until inflammation is gone.

GOTU KOLA TEA

Add 2 teaspoons of dried gotu kola leaves to 1 cup of boiling water. Cover and steep 10 to 15 minutes. Sweeten with honey, if desired. Drink several cups daily.

COUCH GRASS
Agropyron repens (Triticum repens)

OTHER NAMES: Dog grass, durfa grass, witchgrass, wheatgrass, quick grass, twitch grass.
PART USED: Root and rhizomes.
SIGNATURE: The smooth roots have the ability to penetrate the root system of larger, sturdier plants.

Present in the herb are carotene, inulin, glucose, polysaccharides, and vitamin C.

Couch grass has been used for centuries in treating genitourinary-tract disorders. It helps relieve prostate problems because it eliminates gravel and stones from the bladder and kidneys and helps reduce uncontrollable urination. The herb is especially useful for burning and frequent urination.

Couch grass lessens the pain of bladder irritation. Used extensively for enlargement of the prostate, the herb has blood-purifying properties and is a good tonic for the liver and spleen. It is most often used as a tincture.

Caution: While it can be used to relieve urine retention, couch grass should NOT be used for the kidneys if blood is present. Use the herb horsetail (*Equisetum arvense*) instead.

GONORRHEA TREATMENT

Prepare tinctures of couch grass, motherwort, sandalwood, buchu leaves, and saw palmetto by adding 2 tablespoons of each herb to separate pint jars. Pour 1 cup of vodka over each herb. Close the containers and place them in a warm spot for at least two weeks. Strain and bottle each in separate containers. The recommended dosage is 5 to 20 drops of couch grass tincture, 10 to 15 drops of motherwort tincture, 10 to 15 drops of sandalwood tincture, and 10 to 20 drops of buchu leaf tincture.

For a tea, add the suggested number of drops for the tincture desired to 1 cup of warm water and drink three to four times daily.

ENLARGED PROSTATE BLEND

10 to 15 drops of couch grass tincture
4 to 8 drops of saw palmetto tincture
10 to 20 drops of hydrangea root tincture

You can make this tincture by placing 2 tablespoons each of saw palmetto, couch grass, and hydrangea root in a pint jar. Fill the jar with vodka and cover tightly. Place it in a warm and sunny spot for two or more weeks. Strain and pour the mixture into a sterile container. Label with the ingredients, use, and dose. Add 1 to 2 tablespoons of the tincture to 1 cup of hot water. Drink 1 cup morning, noon, and evening as a treatment for an enlarged prostate.

SIBERIAN GINSENG
Eleuthrococcus senticosus

OTHER NAMES: Man's health, five-fingers, sang, ninsin, panax, pannag, red berry.
PART USED: Root, leaves, and bark.
SIGNATURE: This spiny shrub has a carrot-shaped root.

Siberian ginseng root helps regulate blood sugar and stimulates the immune system and the thyroid hormones. It contains thirteen different gineosides (triterpene saponins), panacaene, b-elemene, panaximol, pectin, choline, simple sugars, bioflavonoids, and traces of germanium.

It has vitamins A, B_1, and B_{12}, along with selenium, phosphorus, cobalt, calcium, camphor, iron, magnesium, manganese, and potassium. It stimulates and strengthens the adrenocortical system. It also stimulates the male sex glands. Siberian ginseng contains properties that increase production of RNA and DNA. It is also used as a mild sedative.

For centuries, both men and women have used ginseng as a tonic. It acts as a whole-body tonic that provides extra energy. Combining ginseng with parsley works as a corrective combination for men to relieve swelling and inflammation of the kidneys and prostate. It can be used specifically for treatment of prostatitis.

Caution: People with hypoglycemia, high blood pressure, or heart disease must avoid Siberian ginseng.

SIBERIAN GINSENG–PARSLEY TEA

Mix 1 teaspoon each of chopped ginseng root and finely chopped, fresh parsley. Place the herbs in a cup and pour 1 cup of boiling water over them. Cover and steep 15 minutes. Strain and drink several times daily.

PROSTATE TONIC

> 1 tablespoon of Siberian ginseng root
> 1 tablespoon of goldenseal
> 1 tablespoon of bearberry (uva ursi)
> 1 tablespoon of black cohosh
> 1 tablespoon of wild yam

Place the herbs in a pint jar and fill the jar with vodka or brandy. Allow the mixture to sit for at least two weeks in a sunny window. Strain and place in a sterile container. The dosage recommended is $1/2$ dropper under the tongue several times daily.

DAMIANA
Turnera diffusa

PART USED: Leaves.

Damiana contains chlorophyll, volatile oils, damianian, resin, arbutin, calcium, chromium, cobalt, iron, phosphorus, selenium, silicon, magnesium, manganese, zinc, and vitamins A, B_1, B_3, and C. According to Aztec legends, damiana was used as a powerful aphrodisiac. The volatile oils act as a strong diuretic. The herb is a blood purifier with many of the same components as juniper berries and parsley. It helps relieve many forms of impotence. It contains beta-sitosterol and other aromatic oils that stimulate and regenerate hormonal health. It's fine to use on a regular basis because it enriches the entire genitourinary system. It promotes sexual health.

Caution: Damiana can interfere with iron absorption.

DAMIANA TEA

For a tea, the recommended dose is 1 teaspoon of the herb to 1 cup of boiling water. Drink several cups per day. If using the capsules, take 2 #00 capsules twice daily.

DAMIANA TINCTURE

Place 1 tablespoon of damiana leaves and 1 tablespoon of black cohosh in a pint jar. Pour $1\frac{1}{2}$ cups of vodka over the herbs and cover tightly. Place the jar in a sunny window for two weeks. Strain and place the tincture in a sterile container. Use 1 teaspoon of the tincture to 1 cup of hot water or tea. Take 2 to 3 cups daily.

DAMIANA CAPSULES

> 1 tablespoon of powdered damiana leaves
> 1 tablespoon of powdered saw palmetto
> 1 tablespoon of powdered licorice root
> 1 tablespoon of powdered kelp

Mix the herbs well and fill #00 capsules. Take 2 to 4 capsules daily.

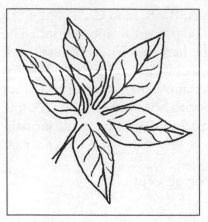

Pau d'Arco

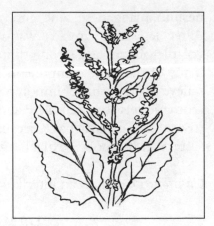

Yellow Dock

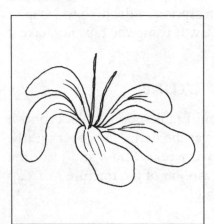

Plantain

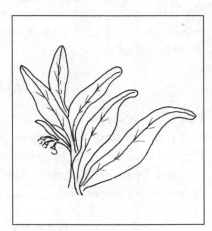

Comfrey

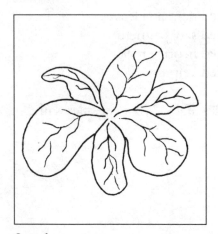

Sorrel

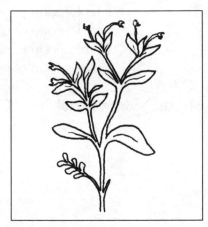

Chickweed

7. Cancer

Early detection is important in any treatment of cancer. Four main types of cancer are lymphomas, carcinomas, sarcomas, and leukemia. Every minute, someone dies from cancer. Over 3 million Americans suffer from this disorder, and of the people who develop cancer, one in three will die. The major causes of cancer are thought to be diet, environment, and stress. Many environmental and dietary carcinogens are being discovered in laboratories worldwide. Experts from the U.S. Environmental Protection Agency have stated that pesticides, diffused in the air and infecting the soil of farmlands and part of the food we eat, are one of the top three environmental cancer risks.

Some scientists believe an excess of iron in the body increases the risk of developing cancer. Take no iron supplements if you have cancer. The cancer-killing function of macrophages and the B-cells and T-cells can be affected if excess iron is present.

Increased calcium intake, according to *The New England Journal of Medicine,* may help prevent precancer cells from becoming malignant. Also, over 200 scientists around the globe have found that vitamin B_3 (niacin) is effective in preventing and treating cancerous growth. Lung cancer, more frequent in the male population, appears to be linked to beta-carotene and vitamins A and E deficiencies.

Obesity appears to play a part in the development of uterine cancer. And overweight women with breast cancer do not respond well to treatment. Breast cancer has also been linked to an iodine deficiency. Overweight men have an increased risk of developing colon and rectal cancer.

In a 1989 issue of the *Medical Tribune,* men who have had a vasectomy were reported to be three times more likely to develop prostate cancer than the general population. We now believe that it takes as long as twenty years for intestinal cancer to develop, and this is probably the result of a long-standing faulty diet.

Cancer Symptoms

Cancer symptoms are many. Be aware of any changes in your body or bodily functions. Consult a physician immediately if you have any of these symptoms.

Mouth and Throat Cancer: Chronic sore throat, tongue, or mouth or ulcer in the throat, tongue, or mouth that does not heal.

Skin Cancer: Warts that change color or size, flat sores or lesions that resemble moles, any lump under the skin that develops unexpectedly.

Cancer of the Larynx: Hoarseness or persistent cough.

Lung Cancer: Persistent cough and blood in the sputum; persistent chest pain.

Stomach Cancer: Pain or indigestion after eating.

Breast Cancer: Any physical change in the breast, a lump or thickening of breast tissue. Check your breasts monthly for any changes.

Colon Cancer: Any change from normal bowel function, diarrhea or constipation, blood in the stool, rectal bleeding.

Bladder or Kidney Cancer: Frequent urination with blood present in the urine.

Cervical or Uterine Cancer: Unusual discharge, excessive bleeding during menstrual period, bleeding between periods, painful menstrual cycles.

Prostate Cancer: Weak or interrupted flow during urination, continuous pain in the upper thighs, pain in the lower back or pelvis, blood in the urine.

Ovarian Cancer: Often no symptoms appear until the cancer has progressed to a later stage.

Testicular Cancer: Collection of fluids in the scrotum, a thickening or enlargement of the scrotum, mild ache in the groin or lower abdomen, discomfort or pain in the testicle(s) or scrotum, enlargement and tenderness of the breasts.

Leukemia: Fatigue, repeated infections, easy bruising, paleness, weight loss, frequent nosebleeds. Children are most often affected.

Cancer Prevention

The best way to fight cancer is with prevention. Practice the many ways we have to increase our chances of being cancer-free. We need to stay away from certain chemicals, like garden pesticides, cleaning agents, and paints as well as beauty aids like lotions, shampoos, hair sprays, hair dyes, nail polish, and some makeup. The skin acts like a third kidney, absorbing the many substances we place on it. Unnatural substances, like synthetic nonfood chemicals, are difficult for the body to get rid of. The body often stores these foreign chemicals in organs like the liver. Most natural, edible, plant-based substances we ingest can be eliminated by the body if they are not needed or used. Of course, poisons also exist in the plant world, but they are not usually part of the human diet.

Diet plays an important role in your health. You may want to eliminate or lower your intake of many foods that could have a negative impact on your health.

FOODS TO AVOID

White flour, refined flours, and related products
Sugar and related products
Saturated fats
Hot dogs, lunch meats, cured meats like bacon, smoked meats
All processed foods
Salt (Use kelp powder as a substitute.)
Alcohol
Coffee and teas, except herbal teas
Restrict milk products except fresh, whole, unprocessed milk.
Reduce intake of meat products.
Limit soybean products since they inhibit enzyme production.

FOODS TO EAT

Eat all the fresh, organically grown vegetables you desire. Juices are important and very helpful. Drink fruit juices in the morning and vegetable juices in the afternoon. Drink apple juice daily since it helps remove toxins from the body. Also, all dark juices, like black currant, beet, grape, blackberry, and black cherry appear helpful. These combination vegetable juices are recommended: cabbage and carrot, carrot and asparagus, or carrot and celery. Eat at least ten raw almonds daily since they are high in laetrile, a well-known cancer treatment.

OTHER FOODS TO EAT

Grains	Seeds	Garlic	Chickpeas
Peas	Dark-Green Vegetables	High-Fiber Cereals	Red Beans
Yams	Millet	Beans	Fish
Wheat	Brussels Sprouts	Chicken	Bran
Broccoli	Brown Rice	Oats	Cauliflower
Whole-Grain Bread	Nuts	Cabbage	Berries
Grapes	Carrots	Apples	Squash
Plums	Pumpkin	Cantaloupe	Beets
Beet Juice	Onions	Cherries	Asparagus

RECOMMENDED NUTRIENTS

As a treatment for cancer, it is also important to add these nutrition supplements to your daily diet for at least three months: beta-carotene, vitamins A, B complex, plus extra B_3, C, and E; calcium, magnesium, selenium, kelp, and garlic.

Beta-carotene: Take 10,000 IU of this strong antioxidant daily.

Vitamin A: Take from 50,000 to 100,000 IU daily for ten days.

Vitamin E: Take 1,000 IU daily.

Vitamin B Complex: Take 100 mg daily.

Vitamin C: Begin with 1,000 mg and slowly build up to a higher dosage of 5,000 to 10,000 mg. Gradually reduce your dosage the same way you began.

Vitamin B_3 (niacin): Take 100 mg daily of this vitamin which helps build red blood cells.

Calcium: Take 2,000 mg daily.

Magnesium: Take 1,000 mg daily.

Selenium: Take 200 mcg of this powerful antioxidant, which is concentrated in the liver, pituitary gland, and pancreas.

Kelp: Take 5 to 8 tablets daily for mineral balance.

Garlic: Take 2 capsules three times daily. You can use the odorless variety.

Consult the lists in chapter 10 for good food and herb sources of these nutrients. Eat and ingest suggested foods and herbs in addition to taking these nutritional supplements if you are fighting cancer.

HELPFUL HERBS

These herbs are helpful in the treatment of cancer: dandelion, burdock, pau d'arco, red clover, plantain, sorrel, yellow dock, ginseng, chickweed, and comfrey. Recipes suggest ways for using these herbs singly or in combination.

Also, tumors respond well to cold-pressed castor oil or to bloodroot (*Sanguinaria canadensis*), applied in a poultice. Soak a flannel cloth with the oil and apply warm to the area where needed. Cover the cloth with a piece of plastic and place a heating pad over the poultice. Apply for at least a half-hour daily.

DANDELION
Taraxacum officinale

OTHER NAMES: Blowball, lion's tooth, wild endive, common dandelion, cankerwort.
PART USED: Root, leaves, and flowers.
SIGNATURE: The yellow flower is the herb's signature.

Dandelion is native to Greece, but it is found in virtually every country in the world. Gather the root when the plant is flowering. Per ounce, the root contains 14,000 IU of vitamin A, which acts as an antioxidant that reacts with carcinogens to make them into harmless substances. Dandelions are also a high source of vitamins B, C, and E, and bioflavonoids. The plant also contains inulin, calcium, protein, phosphorus, selenium, magnesium, potassium, and silicon. Dandelion is used mainly as a blood purifier. It destroys acids in the blood and strains and filters toxins in the bloodstream.

Its stimulation of bile production and liver function encourages elimination of toxins in the blood. It benefits the spleen and improves the health of the pancreas. The herb also builds the immune system and is a good all-around tonic.

113

The leaves can be cooked as a potherb or added to salads. The roots are often used as a coffee substitute with the addition of chicory root. The blossoms make a delicious jelly.

DANDELION LEAF TEA

Use the green leaves. Place 5 to 6 bruised fresh leaves in a cup. Pour boiling water over them and cover the cup. Steep 15 minutes. Strain and drink as many cups per day as desired.

DANDELION ROOT INFUSION

Place 1 ounce of chopped fresh root in a quart jar. Cover the herb with cold water and screw on lid. Allow the mixture to steep overnight. Strain and store in the refrigerator; drink cold throughout the day. Make fresh daily.

DANDELION ROOT TEA

Add 1 to 2 teaspoons of chopped root to 1 cup of boiling water. Cover and steep 30 minutes. Drink cold at meals.

DANDELION TINCTURE

Put 2 ounces of dried chopped dandelion root in a quart jar. Fill the jar with vodka and screw on lid. Allow the jar to stand in a very warm area or sunny window for at least two weeks. Shake occasionally. Strain and place in a sterile bottle. As a tonic or treatment, take several drops to several full droppers daily, depending on need. The tincture can be added to juice or any tea.

BURDOCK
Arctium lappa

OTHER NAMES: Lappa minor, thorny burr, lappa, beggar's-buttons, burs, clotbur, great burdock, edible burdock, cuckold, harlock.
PART USED: Roots, seeds, and leaves.
SIGNATURE: The seeds, the color of the stalk, and the shape of the flower head are burdock's signature.

Burdock has long been used as an alterative or blood cleanser. Burdock slowly improves the health of the body and blood with its nutritional benefits. It enhances liver function. The herb is also a diuretic and a diaphoretic. Through these three actions it removes toxins from the body.

It has antibiotic and antifungal properties. Burdock works as both a cancer preventive and a remedy. Its bacteriostatic properties, due to polyolefins in its volatile oils, inhibit tumor growth. The herb balances the intestinal flora. Since burdock is rich in minerals it can replace those lost during the blood-cleansing process.

It contains calcium, potassium, selenium, protein, magnesium, manganese, phosphorus, cobalt, silicon, sodium, copper, inulin, biotin, and vitamins A, B_1, B_2, B_3, B_6, B_{12}, and E.

Used as a tonic or treatment, it stimulates the immune system. Burdock is an ingredient found in Essiac, a standard alterative treatment for cancer. The tops, gathered before flowering and stripped of the rind, taste similar to asparagus.

Caution: Burdock root interferes with iron absorption.

BURDOCK TINCTURE

Place $1/2$ ounce of burdock root and $1/2$ ounce of dandelion root in a quart jar. Fill the jar with vodka and cover. Allow the mixture to stand at least two weeks in a sunny window. Shake occasionally. Strain and place the contents in a sterile jar. Take 8 to 20 drops in tea or juice twice daily, morning and evening.

BURDOCK CAPSULES

1 tablespoon of powdered red beet
1 tablespoon of powdered yellow dock
1 tablespoon of powdered burdock root

Mix the powdered herbs and fill #00 capsules. Take 2 to 6 capsules daily for three months.

COMBINATION CANCER TREATMENT

The ingredients in this cancer treatment, pau d'arco, yellow dock, dandelion, and burdock, do not have to be powdered. To make the tea, simply mix together 1 tablespoon each of these herbs. Use 1 teaspoon of the herb mixture to 1 cup of boiling water poured over the herbs. Steep 10 minutes and strain; use honey as a sweetener, if desired.

To prepare the capsules, mix 1 tablespoon of each of the powdered herbs and fill #00 capsules. Take 2 to 6 capsules daily.

For a tincture, use 1 tablespoon each of the powdered herbs and steep in 1 quart of vodka or brandy for two weeks in a sunny window. Take 1 teaspoon daily.

PAU D'ARCO
Tabebuia heptaphylla

OTHER NAMES: Taheebo, lapacho, ipe.
PART USED: Inner bark.
SIGNATURE: The red, pink, or violet flowers (although the violet leaves of the tree are said to be the most useful) are the signature. The red flowers indicate blood-cleansing properties.

Pau d'arco has sixteen known naphthaquinones, along with other unknown factors, that produce antitumor effects. Purified naphthaquinones in studies had little antitumor effects, but the unpurified product produced the desired results. Natives from the West Indies, Central America, and South America have used it extensively as a cancer cure. The cure consisted of a tea brewed from the inner bark. Pau d'arco contains antifungal and antibacterial properties along with antimalarial and antibiotic compounds. It is said to cure leukemia.

Pau d'arco contains sitosterol saponins, chrysophanic acid, fixed oils, and resin. The minerals present are calcium, phosphorus, potassium, magnesium, cobalt, chromium, and it contains vitamins A and C.

PAU D'ARCO TEA

Place ½ ounce of pau d'arco in a pan and add 1 quart of water. Simmer for a ½ hour. Strain and drink the tea warm several times daily. Use honey to sweeten, if desired.

PAU D'ARCO SYRUP

Prepare the tea as above with the water and herb. Strain and measure. Add an equal amount of honey or sugar. Bring the mixture to a boil and cook until a syrup is formed. This should take about 10 minutes. Remove from heat and store in a sterile container. Refrigerate. Take 1 tablespoon several times daily. This syrup can be used to sweeten other teas.

PAU D'ARCO POULTICE

Pau d'arco can be used as a poultice for external skin cancers and tumors. Prepare it as a tea, using the powdered herb, and soak a cloth in the tea. Place the cloth on the affected area and keep it warm. Replace frequently. You can also place the herb from the tea inside the cloth, fold the cloth over, and soak the cloth in the tea. Place the cloth on the area, and put a dry towel over it. Then place a heating pad over the poultice. Use the poultice several times daily for at least $^1/_2$ hour. Continue as long as it's needed.

PAU D'ARCO CAPSULES

2 tablespoons of powdered pau d'arco
1 tablespoon of powdered yellow dock
1 tablespoon of powdered dandelion root
1 tablespoon of powdered ginseng

Mix the herbs and fill #00 capsules. Take 2 to 8 capsules daily for up to three months.

RED CLOVER
Trifolium pratense

OTHER NAMES: Cow grass, purple clover, trefoil, cleaver grass.
PART USED: Flowering tops.
SIGNATURE: The red blossoms are its signature.

Red clover, a member of the pea family, is rich in minerals. It is used as an alterative or blood purifier. The herb is antibiotic in nature and has been used as a treatment for AIDS. It has also been used extensively in folk remedies as a cure for tumors and cancers. When added to chaparral, it reduces tumors. Red clover is added to Essiac remedy as a nutritive support for the system. High in minerals, it contains copper, glycosides, magnesium, manganese, selenium, calcium, cobalt, phosphorus, potassium, silicon, sodium, and zinc. It also has coumaric acid, coumestrol, saponins, salicylic acid, and salicylate. The flavonoids present contain estrogenic and antispasmodic properties. Red clover has antibiotic action against several bacteria, especially the pathogen that causes tuberculosis.

The vitamins present are A, B_1, B_2, B_3, B_5, B_9, B_{12}, C, and biotin. Use the plant as a potherb and add to salads.

RED CLOVER TEA

Add 1 to 2 tablespoons of the fresh blossom or 1 to 2 teaspoons of the dried blossoms to 1 cup of boiling water. Cover and steep for 10 to 15 minutes. Strain and drink with every meal.

RED CLOVER CAPSULES

1 tablespoon of powdered red clover
1 tablespoon of powdered pau d'arco
1 tablespoon of powdered echinacea root or leaves
1 tablespoon of powdered blessed thistle

Mix the powdered herbs and fill #00 capsules. Take 6 to 10 capsules daily for several weeks.

RED CLOVER–ST.-JOHN'S-WORT

1 tablespoon of Saint-John's-wort
1 tablespoon of red clover

Place 2 teaspoons of the herb mixture in a cup. Pour 1 cup of boiling water over the herbs and steep for 15 minutes. Strain and add honey if desired. Drink several cups daily.

RED CLOVER TINCTURE

Place 1 ounce of red clover blossoms in a quart jar. Cover the herb completely with vodka and close tightly. Allow it to stand in a warm sunny window for at least two weeks. Strain and place in a sterile bottle. Add 1 teaspoon to tea, juice, or water, and drink.

PLANTAIN
Plantago major

OTHER NAMES: White-man's-foot, cochoo's bread, Englishman's foot, ribwort, wagbread, ripplegrass, snakeweed, cart-track plant.
PART USED: Leaves and root.
SIGNATURE: Flowering spikes are the signature.

Plantain stimulates the immune system and is used as a treatment for breast cancer, colon cancer, and other cancers of the digestive system. The herb regulates the colonic flora and absorbs toxins from the intestines. It is also an alterative or blood cleanser.

Native Americans used plantain to heal chronic sores. Ancient Greek, Roman, Arabian, and Persian physicians also valued plantain for its healing properties.

The herb contains calcium, magnesium, phosphorus, potassium, protein, selenium, silicon, and zinc. Also present are vitamins B_3, C, and K, and factor T, which stops bleeding.

PLANTAIN OINTMENT

Place 2 ounces of plantain in a stainless-steel pan, and pour $1/2$ pint of vegetable oil over the herb. Bring the mixture to a slow simmer and simmer for about 2 hours. Strain after it has cooled. If coconut oil is used the oil will harden somewhat after cooling. If desired, bring the oil just to warm and add melted beeswax to it. Test the consistency by placing a spoon coated with the oil mixture in the refrigerator. If it's too hard, add a little more warm oil; if too soft, add a little more melted beeswax. The ointment should be the consistency of a salve. As a preservative, add several drops of vitamin E oil or several teaspoons of honey. Both are preservatives as well as healers.

PLANTAIN POULTICE

Use a poultice to treat external sores or cancers. Place 1 quart of water in a stainless-steel pan. Add several ounces of plantain to the water. Simmer for about 15 minutes. Dip a cloth into the resulting tea and wring it out slightly. Place some of the herbs from the liquid onto the cloth and fold it over. Place the cloth on the area needed and put a heating pad over a dry, thin towel on the poultice. Use this poultice at least twice daily. Between poultices, wash the area with the tea.

PLANTAIN-BUGLEWEED TEA

1 tablespoon of plantain
1 tablespoon of bugleweed
1 tablespoon of goldenseal

Mix the herbs and place 1 teaspoon of the mixture in a cup. Pour 1 cup of boiling water over the herbs and steep 15 minutes. Drink with meals.

COLON CANCER TEA

$\frac{1}{2}$ ounce of marshmallow
$\frac{1}{2}$ ounce of plantain
$\frac{1}{2}$ ounce of ginseng

As a treatment for colon cancer make this tea. Place the herbs in a stainless-steel pan and add 2 quarts of water. Bring to a quick boil and remove from heat immediately. Cover and steep until cool. Strain and place the mixture in a sterile container. Drink cold several times daily.

PLANTAIN TINCTURE

To get the needed properties on a daily basis, you could make the plantain into a tincture. Add 1 ounce of plantain to a quart jar. Fill the jar with vodka or brandy. Steep at least two weeks in a warm area. Strain and pour the tincture in a sterile bottle. Take 1 tablespoon of the tincture in a cup of hot water, or add it to other herbal teas or juice.

SORREL
Rumex acetosa

OTHER NAMES: Meadow sorrel, garden sorrel, redtop sorrel, sour dock, French sorrel.
PART USED: Leaves.
SIGNATURE: Red pigment in the root, often found in the leaves, is the signature.

Sorrel is a major ingredient of the Essiac cancer treatment. The herb contains potassium, calcium, phosphorus, iodine, sulfur, chlorine, sodium, copper, magnesium, manganese, and citric, oxalic, and malic acids. Vitamins A, B complex, C, D, and E are also present.

Sorrel leaves are used as a potherb and in salads. Sorrel can be used internally and externally as a cancer treatment.

SORREL POULTICE

Add 6 ounces of the sorrel to 2 quarts of water. Bring to a slow simmer and simmer for 15 minutes. Remove from heat and cool. Dip a cloth into the tea. Place some of the sorrel on the area needed and place the cloth over the area. Put a heating pad over the poultice, and allow the treatment to continue for at least a $1/2$ hour several times daily.

SORREL TEA

Make fresh tea by chopping a sorrel leaf and placing it into a cup. Pour 1 cup boiling water over the herb and cover. Steep 15 minutes. Drink with every meal.

COLD SORREL TEA

Place several ounces of sorrel in a pan and pour several cups of boiling water over it. Allow the tea to stand until cool, covered. Strain and refrigerate. Drink several small glasses per day as a treatment for any cancer.

YELLOW DOCK
Rumex crispus

OTHER NAMES: Narrow dock, sour dock, garden patience, rumex, curled dock.
PART USED: Top of plant and root.
SIGNATURE: The color of the root and the lance-shape leaves are yellow dock's signature.

Yellow dock is used mainly as a tonic for the liver. Since the liver filters toxins, its health is very important. Yellow dock aids colon function. It is a good blood purifier that tones the whole system.

Yellow dock is an astringent, alterative, laxative, and it is antimicrobial and fights scurvy. It tones lymph and other glands. Tumors can be treated internally and externally with yellow dock. The herb is often used to treat cancer of the lung and bowels. This Eurasian plant is a close relative of sorrel (*Rumex acetosa*).

The leaves can be used as a potherb. Boil them, discard the water, and boil them again.

Yellow dock contains calcium, magnesium, manganese, niacin, phosphorus, potassium, protein, rumicin, riboflavin, sodium, and tin. It is also high in vitamins A and C and has many trace minerals. That's why it is used as a nutritive tonic.

YELLOW DOCK POULTICE FOR HARD TUMORS

Apply the bruised yellow-dock root to the area needed. Cover and allow the poultice to stay on at least $1/2$ hour. Many people place the root on the problem area, with a bandage covering the root, and leave it overnight.

YELLOW DOCK SYRUP

Place 1 pound of crushed yellow-dock root into a stainless-steel pan. Pour $1^{1}/_{2}$ pints of syrup of any kind over the herb. Bring to a simmer and simmer for 1 hour. Remove from heat and strain. Place in a sterile bottle and refrigerate. Take 1 tablespoon of syrup daily.

YELLOW DOCK TEA

Add $1/2$ cup of chopped yellow root to 2 pints of water. Bring to a boil and reduce heat immediately to simmer for 15 minutes. Strain and place in a sterile container. Refrigerate and drink $1/2$ cup, morning and evening.

YELLOW DOCK OINTMENT

Add $1/2$ ounce of chopped yellow-dock root to 1 pint of coconut oil. Simmer for $1/2$ hour. Strain and apply to external tumors or sores.

YELLOW DOCK CAPSULES

> 1 tablespoon of powdered yellow dock
> 1 tablespoon of powdered beet
> 1 tablespoon of powdered ginseng

Mix the herbs and fill #00 capsules. Take 2 to 6 capsules daily.

GINSENG
Panax quinquefolius

OTHER NAMES: Man's health, five-fingers, American ginseng, sang, red berry, ninsin, pannag.

SIGNATURE: The ginseng root is in the shape of a human and its berries are red.

Ginseng stimulates the lymph glands. Ginseng is well known for its ability to regenerate and rebuild physical energy. Allow at least $1\frac{1}{2}$ months to regenerate the glands. Ginseng improves blood circulation, increases metabolism, and stimulates the endocrine system. It also strengthens the adrenal glands and enhances immune-system function. It aids liver function by generating new cells.

The herb is a stimulant for the heart, brain, and central nervous system. It corrects adrenal and thyroid function, reduces stress, and strengthens the body to counteract debilitating disease.

Ginseng contains calcium, protein, potassium, phosphorus, magnesium, manganese, sodium, copper, selenium, and fat. Vitamins B_{12}, C, and E are present in ginseng.

GINSENG TEA

Add $\frac{1}{2}$ teaspoon of ginseng to 1 cup of boiling water. Steep for 10 to 15 minutes. Strain and drink several cups per day.

GINSENG CAPSULES

Mix 1 tablespoon each of powdered ginseng and powdered garlic. Fill #00 capsules. Take 2 to 4 capsules daily.

GINSENG COMBINATION CAPSULES

>1 tablespoon of powdered ginseng
>1 tablespoon of powdered licorice root
>1 tablespoon of powdered yellow dock

Mix the herbs and place mixture in #00 capsules. Take 2 to 6 capsules daily.

CHICKWEED
Stellaria media

OTHER NAMES: Scarwort, satin flower, starweed, adder's mouth, stitchwort.

PART USED: Whole top of plant.

Chickweed contains steroidal saponins, biotin, choline, copper, inositol, PABA, phosphorus, rutin, silicon, magnesium, protein, and vitamins B_6, B_{12}, C, and D. It is extremely high in vitamin A. Use the plant as a potherb or as an addition to other foods and salads.

The herb is used as a blood cleanser, and it supplies many needed vitamins and minerals. Chickweed is used as a treatment for colon cancer since it absorbs toxins from the intestines and regulates colonic bacteria and yeast. It is also used to treat cancer of the testes.

CHICKWEED TESTES POULTICE

Place 2 ounces of chickweed in a stainless-steel pan. Pour 1 quart of water over the herb and simmer until the liquid is reduced to $1\frac{1}{2}$ pints. Place the herb on the testes and put a cloth that has been dipped into the tea over the herb. Do this twice daily. Drink the tea daily while using the poultice for prostate or testicular cancer.

CHICKWEED TEA

Place 1 tablespoon of chickweed in a cup. Pour 1 cup of boiling water over the herb. Cover and steep 15 minutes. Strain and drink every two to four hours, if possible.

CANCER CAPSULE REMEDY

Make a capsule by mixing equal parts of chickweed, ginseng, and saw palmetto. You can also mix chickweed, red beet, and yellow dock, if you wish. Place the herb mixture in #00 capsules. Take 2 to 6 capsules daily.

CHICKWEED EXTERNAL SALVE

Place 1 ounce of chickweed in 1 pint of vegetable or coconut oil. Simmer for 20 minutes. Strain and add beeswax, if using vegetable oil, for desired consistency. Coconut oil will harden somewhat after drying. Apply the salve externally to any external cancer.

COMFREY
Symphytum officinale

OTHER NAMES: Healing herb, knitbone, knitback, boneset, gamplant, common comfrey.
PART USED: Leaves and roots.
SIGNATURE: Comfrey has hollow stems, and rough hair covers all parts of the plant. It is thought that this allows the toxins to stick and be flushed from the body.

Comfrey contains sodium, magnesium, manganese, potassium, phosphorus, protein, and vitamins B_1 and B_3. It contains the basic antioxidants vitamins A, C, and E. Comfrey absorbs toxins from the intestines, regulating intestinal flora, so it is useful as a treatment for colon cancer. It is an antiinflammatory, astringent, and hemostat. It aids cell growth. It contains allantoin, tannins, saponins, sitosterol, and alkaloids. Used externally, it soothes skin disorders.

Comfrey may be used as a green drink by placing several leaves in the blender along with orange juice. You can drink this concoction several times weekly. It makes a good blood cleanser.

Caution: When taken internally, comfrey may cause liver damage. Take only under a physician's careful supervision and for a short period. Comfrey is considered safe when used externally as a poultice or an ointment.

COMFREY CAPSULES

Mix together 1 tablespoon each of yellow dock, comfrey, licorice, and plantain. Place the herb mixture in #00 capsules. Take 2 to 4 capsules daily for two months.

COMFREY OINTMENT

Place 1 ounce of plantain and 1 ounce of comfrey root in 1 pint of coconut oil. Simmer for $1/2$ hour. Strain and add several drops of vitamin E oil to the mixture. Use as a salve for external cancers or sores.

COMFREY POULTICE

Place 2 ounces of chopped comfrey root and 2 ounces of chopped burdock root in 1 quart of distilled water. Boil for 15 minutes. Strain the herbs from the liquid and continue boiling until the liquid is halved. Dip a cloth into this tea, and use as a poultice for external cancers and tumors. Change the cloth often.

COMFREY LUNG AND BONE CANCER TREATMENT

An infusion is made by adding 1 teaspoon of comfrey leaves and 1 teaspoon of grated comfrey root. Place the mixture in a cup and add 1 cup of boiling water. Cover and steep 15 minutes. Strain and drink 2 cups daily for two months.

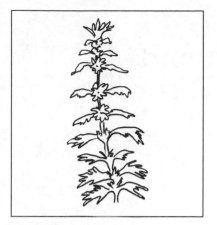

Motherwort

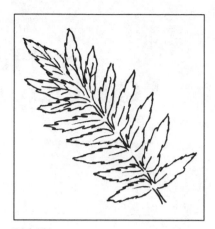

Valerian

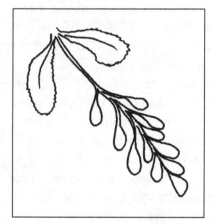

Barberry

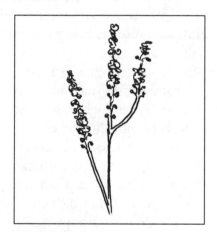

Black Cohosh

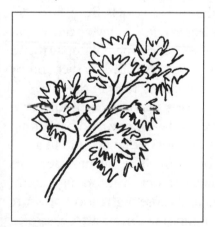

Parsley

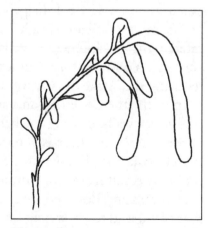

Horsetail

8. Heart and Circulatory Disorders

Cardiovascular disease is the number-one killer in the Western world. Over 50 million Americans suffer from circulatory system disorders and heart disease. Every minute someone dies of a heart attack. About half of all heart-attack victims have no prior symptoms, and one-third of all first-heart-attack sufferers die within the first twenty days.

That's why it's vitally important to take care of the cardiovascular, or circulatory, system, which is made up of the heart and blood vessels. Stress, fatty diet (high cholesterol), smoking, stimulants like coffee and alcohol, oral contraceptives, and inadequate exercise can all contribute to heart disease. They often lead to **hypertension**—what we commonly call high blood pressure. Over 40 million people in the United States alone suffer from hypertension, which can lead to heart failure, stroke, or kidney failure.

Low-density lipoproteins (LDL), so-called bad cholesterol, can cause the bood to clot, while **high-density lipoproteins** (HDL), so-called good cholesterol, help protect the blood vessels from fatty deposits and blood clots. High LDL cholesterol levels have been implicated in the development of gallstones, impotence, mental impairment, and high blood pressure. Cholesterol may be controlled by diet and by reducing the intake of fatty foods while increasing fiber in the diet.

In both atherosclerosis and arteriosclerosis deposits accumulate inside artery walls, causing thickening, reduced elasticity, and hardening of the arteries. In **atherosclerosis,** fatty deposits build up, and in **arteriosclerosis** mostly calcium deposits build up. The calcium deposits probably result from faulty mineral balance rather than too high an intake of calcium. Both reduce circulation and cause high blood pressure that could lead to chest pain on exertion (angina), heart attack, stroke, or sudden cardiac death. Although these fatty or calcium deposits in the arteries cause high blood pressure, the reverse can also be true. And as the arteries become more narrow, blood pressure rises. Cells may experience oxygen starvation because of insufficient circulation as arteries become less pliable and less permeable.

When a coronary artery becomes obstructed by a blood clot or accumulated fatty or calcium deposits, the heart muscle receives less oxygen and the person suffers a heart attack (myocardial infarction), in which the oxygen-starved part of the heart muscle dies, or a coronary occlusion (a coronary). When an artery that supplies the brain with blood and oxygen is occluded, a stroke (cerebrovascular accident) occurs.

Also, **peripheral athcrosclerosis** may affect lower limbs and supply insufficient oxygen. This disease can limit the person's mobility and even lead to loss of a limb. Early signs are aching muscles, fatigue, and cramplike pain in the legs and ankles. If enough oxygen is not getting to the limbs, it's likely that the brain and heart also have diseased arteries.

Symptoms of Heart and Other Cardiovascular Disorders

HEART ATTACK

Myocardial infarction, heart attack, is caused by complete blockage of nutrients and oxygen to the heart. Death of a segment of the heart muscle follows interruption of the heart's supply of blood.

Heart attack symptoms include: (1) prolonged heavy pressure or squeezing pain in the center of the chest behind the sternum. (2) The pain may spread to the neck, shoulder, arm, fourth and fifth fingers of the left hand, back, teeth, or jaw, perhaps accompanied by (3) nausea, (4) sweating, (5) vomiting, and (6) shortness of breath.

These symptoms can come and go. GET IMMEDIATE HELP. It is imperative that the sufferer receive medical care immediately. Death could occur if treatment is not begun at once.

Hypertension symptoms include: (1) dizziness, (2) vision problems, (3) shortness of breath, (4) headache, (5) sweating, and (6) rapid pulse.

Congestive heart disease symptoms are these: (1) fatigue, (2) labored breathing after mild exercise, (3) fluid accumulation, and (4) swelling of feet and ankles.

Ischemic heart disease is caused by arteriosclerosis.

MYOCARDIAL INSUFFICIENCY

Myocardial insufficiency is the term for the heart's inability to perform its usual functions. This leads to cardiac failure.

Angina pectoris is caused by an insufficient supply of blood to the heart. Symptoms may be brief or last for a considerable period of time. **Symptoms** include: (1) Severe pain and constriction about the heart, often radiating down the left arm. Pain may also be felt in the back or jaw. (2) Pressure or severe pain in the area of the heart. (3) Anxiety and fear of approaching death. (4) The face will become pale, livid, or ashen. (5) The pulse generally becomes rapid. (6) Blood pressure will rise. (7) Arrhythmia, or erratic heartbeat, may be present.

Angina vasomotoria involves angina pectoris but with milder **symptoms.** These include: (1) pallor, (2) cyanosis, and (3) coldness and numbness of the hands and feet.

Cardiac arrest involves (1) brief dizziness and (2) loss of consciousness. (3) The heart stops beating.

ARRHYTHMIAS AND HEART PALPITATIONS

Arrhythmias involve disruption of the natural rhythm of the heart.

Cardiac arrhythmia is irregular heartbeat caused by pathological disturbances in the discharge of cardiac electrical impulses from the sino-atrial node or disruption of the transmission of these impulses through the conductile tissue of the heart.

Sinus arrhythmia is cardiac irregularity characterized by increased heart rate. The sinus node of the heart does not initiate impulses for the heartbeat. This has no clinical significance except in older patients, in whom it may indicate coronary artery disease.

Heart palpitations are characterized by the heart beating out of sequence or the heart skipping beats.

SELF-TEST FOR HEART PROBLEMS

Take your pulse first thing in the morning. If the pulse is under 60, your heart is functioning fine. If the pulse is above 80, you may want to consider changes in your lifestyle and diet. If it is consistently above 80, consult your physician.

If you are suffering from **high blood pressure** (hypertension), remember that this condition is a precursor to heart trouble.

Obesity and a sedentary lifestyle, as well as stress, can lead to heart disease. Lack of calcium, usually because of mineral imbalance, has been linked to hypertension.

RECOMMENDED NUTRIENTS FOR HYPERTENSION

If you have hypertension, supplement your daily diet with these vitamins, minerals, and herbs for about three months.

Vitamin B Complex: Take 50 mg three times daily with meals.
Vitamin C: Take 1,000 mg daily with each meal.
Vitamin E: Take 100 IU daily.
Coenzyme Q10:   Take 100 mg daily.
Calcium: Take 1,500 to 3,000 mg daily.
Lecithin: Take 1 to 2 capsules daily.
Magnesium: Take 1,000 mg divided during the day, after meals and before bedtime.
Selenium: Take 200 mcg daily.
Zinc: Take 50 mg daily.
Apple pectin: Use it as a sweetener. Sprinkle it on foods, take it in capsules, or use it any way you can to get it into your body.
Garlic: Take 2 capsules three times daily with meals.
Kelp: Take 6 to 8 capsules daily; kelp is rich in minerals.
Primrose: Take as directed before meals.

A preventive lifestyle and diet is the best treatment for hypertension. A high-fiber diet is also recommended. Avoid a high-fat diet. This means staying away from all animal fat. Eat fish and poultry only. Eliminate caffeine, tobacco, alcohol, sugar, margarine, fats, red meats, fried foods, soft drinks, and white-flour products. Eat raw foods when possible. Also eat onions, garlic, broiled or baked poultry, almonds, olive oil, broiled or baked seafood, and fresh, organically grown vegetables.

Juice is recommended daily. Take fruit juices in the morning and vegetable juices in the afternoon. You can make many mixtures for variety or drink a single juice at a time. This is just a small list.

| Cranberry | Carrot and Celery | Citrus | Beet |
| Watermelon | Spinach | Apple | Cabbage |

HERBS HELPFUL FOR HEART DISEASE

These herbs are recommended for people with heart disease and related ailments: motherwort, cayenne pepper (capsicum), hawthorn berries, barberry, parsley, valerian, ginseng, horsetail, and black cohosh. Consult your physician about using these herbs as a supplement with your prescription medications.

High blood pressure is a silent killer, so you need to eliminate certain foods from your diet and take immediate steps to change your lifestyle. To avoid a high salt intake, it's good to learn how to season with herbs. Many are useful. Avoid taking licorice root, however, since it can disrupt heart function.

MOTHERWORT
Leonurus cardiaca

OTHER NAMES: Lion's tail, lion's ear, throwwort, heart herb.
PART USED: Upper part of the herb.
SIGNATURE: The herb has sharp thorns indicative of sharp pain.

Motherwort improves coronary health and removes congestion and wastes from the body. It also strengthens and improves the central nervous system. It is a member of the mint family. It can be used as a treatment for heart palpitations, heart weakness, and shortness of breath. It lowers and regulates high blood pressure, normalizes heart function, and promotes healthy sleep.

Motherwort is considered a hypotensive, nervine, and antispasmodic. It calms and reduces the risk of thrombosis and stimulates the circulation. It has antibacterial and antifungal properties.

Use motherwort to remove congestion and wastes from the body, and as a treatment for a heart condition and high blood pressure. You can prepare tinctures of motherwort and other herbs.

HERBAL HEART TINCTURES

Place ¹/₂ ounce of motherwort, black cohosh root, and burdock root each in separate pint jars. Finish filling the pints with vodka or brandy. Allow the mixtures to sit in a warm area or sunny window for about two weeks. Shake the jars daily. Strain and place the contents in separate sterile containers. Then prepare a tea.

> 1 tablespoon of motherwort tincture
> 1 tablespoon of black cohosh root tincture
> 2 tablespoons of burdock root tincture

Mix the tinctures. Use 1 teaspoon of this mixture in 1 cup of hot water. Drink twice daily.

MOTHERWORT TEA

Motherwort can be used alone to lower high blood pressure. Add 1 teaspoon of motherwort to 1 cup of boiling water. Allow the tea to steep, covered, for about 15 minutes. Strain and drink with each meal.

MOTHERWORT CAPSULES

> 1 tablespoon of powdered motherwort
> 1 tablespoon of powdered hawthorn berries
> 1 tablespoon of powdered apple pectin

Mix the herbs well and fill #00 capsules. Take 2 capsules three times daily.

CAYENNE PEPPER
Capsicum annum

OTHER NAMES: Capsicum, red pepper, African bird pepper, chili pepper, bird pepper.
PART USED: Fruit.
SIGNATURE: The red fruit or pepper is the signature.

Cayenne pepper (capsicum) is a catalyst for other herbs, but it is also considered the most persistent heart stimulant. It improves circulation. Capsicum works to lower cholesterol by preventing the absorption of cholesterol. It acts in a reflexive way to reduce blood pressure and increase the oxygen-exchange capacity of the lungs while stimulating and promoting cardiovascular activity.

The herb contains capsacutin, capsaicin, capsico, capsanthine, and apsaicine, along with the nutrients PABA, calcium, magnesium, phosphorus, potassium, protein, silicon, manganese, iron, and vitamins A, B_1, B_2, B_3, B_5, B_6, and C.

CAPSICUM CAPSULES

2 teaspoons of capsicum
1 tablespoon of powdered hawthorn berries
1 tablespoon of apple pectin
1 tablespoon of powdered black cohosh

Mix the herbs and fill #00 capsules. Take 2 capsules twice daily.

CAPSICUM COMBINATION CAPSULES

capsicum, parsley, and barberry
or
capsicum, white willow, and valerian
or
capsicum, ginseng, and black cohosh
or
capsicum, motherwort, and garlic
or
capsicum, chickweed, and kelp
or
capsicum, ginseng, and hawthorn

Mix equal parts of any of these powdered herb combinations. Fill #00 capsules. Take 2 to 4 capsules daily.

HAWTHORN BERRIES
Crataegus laevigata (Crataegus oxycantha)

OTHER NAMES: Hagthorn, bread and cheese, English hawthorn, white thorn, quick-set thorn.

PART USED: Berries.

SIGNATURE: The red berries signify use for the blood and for the cardiovascular system.

Active properties isolated in hawthorn berries, crataegin and amygdalin, are now used to lower blood pressure and as a heart tonic. The herb dilates coronary blood vessels, thus lowering blood pressure and cholesterol levels. Hawthorn has long been used to treat heart disease and cardiac arrhythmia, prevent angina pain, and reduce arteriosclerosis. It has antithrombotic action because of the coumarins present. Hawthorn berries also treat high and low blood pressure.

Other components it includes are saponins, tartaric acid, citric acid, cratagolic acid, glavone, and glycosides. The herb is high in potassium, which is good for the heart. It can be taken as a supplement along with a prescription blood pressure drug. But check with your physician first. The herb also contains magnesium, calcium, choline, inositol, PABA, bioflavonoids, and vitamins A, B complex, and C. Take the herb with meals to avoid nausea.

HAWTHORN BERRY CAPSULES

These help lower cholesterol and blood pressure.

> 1 tablespoon of powdered hawthorn berries
> 1 tablespoon of powdered black cohosh root
> 2 teaspoons of cayenne pepper

Mix the herbs and fill #00 capsules. Take 2 to 6 capsules daily with meals.

HAWTHORN-GINKGO TINCTURE

This tincture improves circulation. Place 2 tablespoons each of hawthorn berries and ginkgo in a 1 pint jar. Fill the container with vodka or brandy. Allow it to stand two weeks in a sunny window or in a warm area. Shake daily. Strain and place the contents in a sterile container. Take 1 teaspoon of the tincture in 1 cup of hot water three times daily with meals. The hot water will reduce the alcohol content.

BEET CAPSULES

1 tablespoon of powdered beet root
1 tablespoon of powdered chickweed
1 tablespoon of powdered hawthorn berries

Mix the herbs and fill #00 capsules. Take 2 to 4 capsules three times daily.

HAWTHORN BERRY TEA

Place 2 to 4 teaspoons of crushed hawthorn berries in 1 cup of boiling water. Allow the tea to steep 15 minutes, covered. Strain and drink with every meal.

BARBERRY
Berberis vulgaris

OTHER NAMES: Piprage, berberry, sourberry, jaundice berry.
PART USED: Berries, bark, and root.
SIGNATURE: The red berries and the yellow root are the signature.

Barberry decreases the heart rate and depresses breathing. Use it as a heart tonic. It contains citric and malic acids, oxycanthine, hydrastine, berberrubine, berberine, columbamine, palmatine, and berbamine. It also has calcium, cobalt, iron, magnesium, manganese, potassium, and tin. Barberry contains some of the same alkaloids as goldenseal. These alkaloids constrict capillary blood flow, lower blood pressure, and mobilize the white blood cells of the immune system. The herb increases circulation and has other stimulating effects. It protects the body from scurvy and the blood from metabolic waste. Barberry is also considered an antibiotic, astringent, antifungal, sedative, and antispasmodic.

Caution: Avoid barberry during pregnancy.

BARBERRY TINCTURE

Add 2 tablespoons of crushed barberry to 1 pint of vodka or brandy. Steep two weeks in a warm or sunny area. Strain and bottle in a sterile container. Add 1 teaspoon of the tincture to 1 cup of hot water. Drink three times daily with meals and before going to bed.

BARBERRY CAPSULES

1 tablespoon of powdered barberry
1 tablespoon of powdered ginseng
1 tablespoon of powdered ginger

Mix the herbs and fill #00 capsules. Take 2 capsules three times daily with meals.

BARBERRY TEA

Place 1 to 2 teaspoons of crushed berries in 1 cup of boiling water. Steep 15 minutes, covered. Strain and drink 3 to 4 cups daily.

PARSLEY
Petroselinum crispum

OTHER NAMES: Garden parsley, rock parsley, parsley breakstone, rock selinum.
PART USED: Whole herb, seeds, and root.
SIGNATURE: The yellow flowers are the signature.

Parsley is used for fluid retention and edema. Parsley is diuretic in nature and this makes it hypotensive. Its essential oils are responsible for these actions. The herb is also antimicrobial and a stimulant.

Parsley contains chlorophyll; the chlorophyll molecule includes magnesium. Parsley also contains calcium, potassium, phosphorus, protein, iron, iodine, and vitamins A, B_6, B_{12}, and C. The chemical content is flavone glycoside, petroselinic acid, pinene, myristicene, volatile and essential oils, furanocumarin bergapten, and parsley camphor (apiin). It is best used fresh since chlorophyll oxidizes quickly when dried.

Parsley, cultivated since antiquity, is a valued medicinal herb. Here its most important use is as a diuretic. Parsley, when eaten, has the added benefit of deodorizing garlic.

PARSLEY TEA

Place several tablespoons of chopped parsley in a cup. Pour 1 cup of boiling water over the herb and cover. Allow the tea to steep 15 minutes before straining. Take 2 to 4 cups one day a week for a three-month period. This is a strong diuretic. Be careful; you do not want to overuse the tea since it could deplete the system of much-needed potassium.

PARSLEY CAPSULES

1 tablespoon of powdered parsley
1 tablespoon of powdered Irish moss
1 tablespoon of powdered garlic

Mix the herbs and fill #00 capsules. Take 2 to 4 capsules daily.

PARSLEY TEA OR CAPSULE MIXTURES

dong quai, ginger, and parsley
or
barberry, dandelion, and parsley
or
American ginseng, chickweed, and parsley

To make tea, mix 1 tablespoon of each of the three herbs from the chosen combination above. Add 1 teaspoon of the herb mixture to a cup. Pour 1 cup of boiling water over the herb mixture and cover. Steep 15 minutes, strain, and drink.

To prepare the capsules, mix 1 tablespoon each of the chosen herbs, and fill #00 capsules. Take 2 to 6 capsules per day.

VALERIAN ROOT
Valeriana officinalis

OTHER NAMES: Phu, setwall, great wild valerian, capon's tail, common valerian, garden heliotrope.
PART USED: Root system.
SIGNATURE: The root system is said to resemble the human brain.

Valerian has the highest amount of calcium of any known herb. Calcium is very important to a healthy heart. Valerian is considered a nervine first, but it is also an antispasmodic, antibacterial, anodyne, stimulant, and hypotensive. This diuretic is helpful for kidney disorders, and it is used extensively to lower blood pressure. It suppresses and regulates the autonomic nervous system. The herb has been in use since the 11th century.

Valerian long been used to lower blood pressure, increase heart action, stimulate and improve circulation, and prevent liver necrosis.

The components of valerian are protein, acetic acid, glycosides, camphene, volatile oils, valeric acid, chatinine, pinene, formic acid, and butyric acid. The minerals present are calcium, phosphorus, potassium, tin, iron, magnesium, and a small amount of selenium.

Valerian has a strong odor, and this alone may turn you away from the herb. But valerian is one of the most useful herbs. Your body treats valerian the same way it treats valium, and it is considered one of the most potent sedative herbs. It easily induces sleep for some people. This may be one of the best ways to lower stress levels naturally. Rest is important when working with any disorder and doubly so with hypertension. Here are a few ways you could try valerian.

VALERIAN TINCTURE

Place 1 ounce of valerian in a 1 pint jar, and finish filling the container with vodka or brandy. Place the jar in a warm sunny area for up to a month, depending on the strength desired. Strain and place the tincture in small containers to carry with you. A larger bottle may be useful for storage. Take anywhere from several drops to several full droppers. Start with a lower dosage, and take the herb every fifteen minutes until you see what amount works for you. The effects last about four to five hours. Adjust the dosage at home since valerian may put you to sleep immediately.

Many people who prepare the tincture take it with them to work as an almost instant stress reliever. They add it to juice, water, or tea. You can place the tincture directly under the tongue with a dropper. This allows the herb to go directly into the bloodstream for almost immediate action.

People eventually get used to the taste, and some even come to like it. This herb does so much that the bad taste is worth it. Valerian is also used as an antidote for poison ivy and skin rashes of all sorts. Rub the tincture on the poison ivy rash with a cotton ball. It stops itching immediately. It is also good for hives if placed on the area externally, and it can be taken internally, too. The strength of the odor suggests its potency.

VALERIAN CAPSULES

Some prefer to take valerian in capsules. Capsules take a little longer to work, but they are still effective. Place the herb in #00 capsules and take two, as needed.

Add peppermint in equal amounts to valerian to increase the action of the herb.

VALERIAN COMBINATION CAPSULES

1 tablespoon of powdered valerian
1 tablespoon of powdered white willow
1 tablespoon of powdered black cohosh

Mix the herbs and fill #00 capsules. Take 2 capsules twice daily.

VALERIAN TEA

Many take the herb in tea form after getting used to the taste. Place 1 teaspoon of valerian in a cup. Add 1 cup of boiling water and steep 10 minutes, covered. Strain and drink two times daily. Other herbs can be added if desired for taste.

HORSETAIL
Equisetum hyemale (Equisetum arvense)

OTHER NAMES: Bottlebrush, pewterwort, shavegrass, scouring rush.
PART USED: Top.
SIGNATURE: The plant's unswollen joints and the fact that it grows in wet and gravely places are its signature.

Horsetail increases calcium absorption. It is considered an astringent, antibacterial, and antibiotic. Horsetail also contains the highest amount of silicon of common medicinal herbs.

Native Americans used horsetail grass to treat edema. Horsetail strengthens the heart and lungs. The herb was used as a diuretic for all heart conditions to reduce edema (excess fluids in the tissues), and to improve blood circulation. It is considered a tonic for the whole cardio-vascular system.

Horsetail contains equisitine, fluorine, fatty acids, nicotine, aconitic acid, silica, saponins, and alkaloids. The minerals and vitamins present are zinc, calcium, copper, magnesium, phosphorus, potassium, silicon, iron, aluminum, tin, bioflavonoids, PABA, and vitamins A, B_3, B_5, and C.

HORSETAIL TEA

Place 1 to 2 teaspoons of crushed horsetail herb in a cup. Pour 1 cup of boiling water over the herb and cover. Steep 45 minutes. Take a mouthful of tea several times throughout the day.

HORSETAIL CAPSULES

1 tablespoon of powdered horsetail
1 tablespoon of powdered plantain
1 tablespoon of powdered saw palmetto berries

Mix the powdered herbs and fill #00 capsules. Take 2 capsules morning and evening.

HORSETAIL DIURETIC TEA

1 tablespoon of chopped horsetail
1 tablespoon of chopped dandelion root
1 tablespoon of chopped parsley

Pour 1 quart of boiling water over the chopped herbs, and allow the herb mixture to stand until cool. Strain and place in refrigerator. Drink $1/2$ cup of it cold three times daily for about three days.

HORSETAIL TONIC CAPSULES

1 tablespoon of powdered horsetail
1 tablespoon of powdered ginseng
1 tablespoon of powdered black cohosh

Mix the powdered herbs and fill #00 capsules. Take 2 capsules twice daily.

BLACK COHOSH
Cimicifuga racemosa

OTHER NAMES: Black snakeroot, rattleroot, bugbane, rattletop, squawroot.
PART USED: The root.

Black cohosh is considered an antispasmodic. It is used to treat heart palpitations, cardiac asthma, and high blood pressure, and some practitioners consider it safer to use than digitalis. It inhibits vasomotor centers in the central nervous system and depresses the arterial rate. It lowers cholesterol levels and blood pressure.

Present in black cohosh are oleic acid, palmitic acid, cimicifungin, actaeine, isoferulic acid, racemosin, triterpenes, and estrogenic substances. The vitamins and minerals include phosphorus, potassium, sulfur, magnesium, and vitamins A and B_5.

Caution: Black cohosh should not be used during pregnancy or for chronic disease.

BLACK COHOSH DIURETIC AND HEART TONIC

> 2 ounces of bugleweed
> 3 ounces of walnut leaves
> 1 ounce of chopped black cohosh
> 1 ounce of chopped lily-of-the-valley root
> 2 ounces of crushed hawthorn berries
> 1 ounce of Irish moss

This recipe tones the contractions of the heart and removes fluids from the body. Add the herbs to 1 gallon of distilled water. Bring to a slow boil and reduce heat. Simmer for 20 minutes. Strain the herbs from the liquid, pressing to get all the extracted properties. Return the liquid to the stove and continue simmering until it is reduced to 1 quart. Add 4 pounds of brown sugar and heat thoroughly (about 5 minutes) until the sugar is dissolved, removing scum as it forms. Allow the mixture to stand until lukewarm, and add 1 pint of glycerin. Stir until thoroughly mixed. Pour the mixture into a sterile container and store the tonic in a cool place. Take 1 teaspoon in tea, water, or juice for three days, then take $1/2$ teaspoon for another two days.

HIGH BLOOD PRESSURE REMEDY

1 tablespoon of powdered black cohosh
1 tablespoon of powdered valerian root
1 tablespoon of powdered garlic
2 teaspoons of cayenne pepper

Mix the herbs and fill #00 capsules. Take 2 capsules three times daily for two days. Then reduce the dose to 2 capsules per day for a month.

BLACK COHOSH TEA

This tea reduces blood pressure. Add 1 teaspoon of black cohosh to 1 cup of boiling water. Cover and steep 15 minutes. Drink three times daily with meals for one week out of each month, for three months.

BLACK COHOSH TINCTURE

Add 4 tablespoons of black cohosh to 1 pint of vodka or brandy. Allow the mixture to sit for several weeks in a warm area or sunny window, shaking it daily. Strain and bottle. Take 1 teaspoon of the tincture in 1 cup of hot water daily. Use two days, weekly. To take directly under the tongue, use 1 to 15 drops as a treatment for heart palpitations.

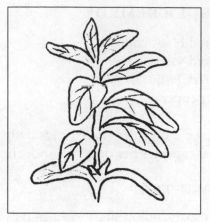

Peppermint

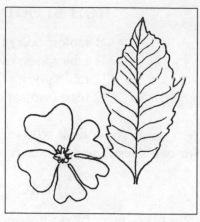

Marshmallow

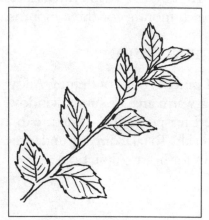

Slippery Elm

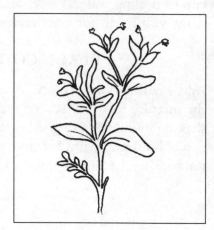

Chickweed

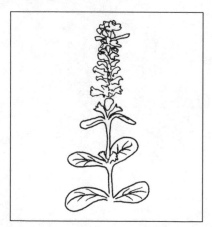

Bugleweed

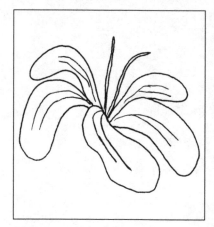

Plantain

9. Intestinal Complaints

Colitis, Crohn's disease, diverticulitis, chronic constipation, and diarrhea are just a few of the problems that can affect your total health. In only about 15 to 20 hours toxins can form from waste in the colon. Keeping the bowel clean is the first step in preventive health. It takes years of eating the wrong foods and not supplying the body with the nutrients necessary for good health before the gastrointestinal system finally breaks down. However, stress also plays an important part in our health. Many intestinal complaints are caused by stress. Once we learn to control our reaction to stress, we reduce the chance that the digestive tract will become a problem.

By giving ourselves the minerals and vitamins we need, we can overcome any imbalance in the body. The healing herbs recommended in this chapter strengthen and support weak tissues because these herbs are composed of balanced natural properties. Your body will respond faster to a natural substance than to synthetics because of the natural balance of phytochemicals and nutrients found in organic sources. Minerals and vitamins are the building blocks of the body and the fuel we need to function properly.

Diet plays the most important role in good health. Those suffering from constipation generally need sodium, chlorine, and magnesium.

Constipation is caused by waste material that stays too long in or moves too slowly through the large intestine. Many disorders result from constipation. Gas, headaches, hernias, insomnia, varicose veins, obesity, hemorrhoids, bad breath, diverticulitis, and colon cancer are just a few. It often takes twenty years of abuse to develop colon cancer.

Many other factors must be considered as well: poor diet, stress, prescription drug reactions, antidepressants, and insufficient fluid and fiber in your daily diet. Food allergies may also be responsible. A test for food allergies may be a good idea if you suffer from any intestinal discomfort.

145

Colitis is an inflammation of the mucous membranes of the colon. There are several types of colitis, ranging from very mild to quite serious symptoms. Small pouchlike sacs are formed in the intestinal wall. Colitis starts with a poor diet, stress, and food allergies. It most often strikes young and middle-aged adults. **Colitis symptoms** include (1) blood in the stool, (2) chronic diarrhea, (3) cramps, (4) feeling a constant need to move the bowels, and (5) gas and bloating.

The disorder at its most severe is usually **ulcerative colitis.** The colon is not simply inflamed but lined with ulcers as well. The symptoms are the same as for ordinary colitis, but much more pronounced.

Enteritis and **ileitis** are inflammations of the small intestine (ileum).

RECOMMENDED NUTRIENTS

Diet plays an important role in the treatment of intestinal complaints. For constipation take sodium, chlorine, and magnesium. Vitamin K helps relieve colitis and other gastrointestinal tract disturbances; a vitamin K supplement or alfalfa liquid daily is helpful.

Also, to treat gastrointestinal system disorders, stay on a high-protein, low-carbohydrate diet. Avoid eating seeds, nuts, grains, sugar products, fried foods, red meats, spices, processed foods, and dairy products, except whole, unpasteurized milk. Take these nutrition supplements.

Vitamin A   Take 25,000 IU daily for tissue repair.
Vitamin B Complex   Take 150 mg in divided doses daily.
Vitamin E   Take 600 IU daily.
Vitamin K or Alfalfa Liquid   Take a 100 mg tablet of vitamin K or 1 tablespoon of alfalfa liquid three times daily.
Kelp   Take 3 tablets of this complex mineral compound, which includes zinc, magnesium, calcium, and chromium.
Acidophilus   Take 3 capsules twice daily on an empty stomach. Acidophilus helps normalize intestinal bacteria.
Proteolytic Enzymes   Take 2 tablets daily between meals.
Multidigestive Enzymes   Take 2 tablets after meals.
Comfrey Pepsin   Take 1 capsule twice daily for $1\frac{1}{2}$ months; check with a physician.
Aloe Vera Juice   Take $\frac{1}{2}$ cup twice daily, morning and evening.

Use a cleansing enema of 2 quarts of warm water daily. For inflammation of the colon, use an enema with lobelia herb tea.

If you have colitis, your diet should include high-fiber foods such as rice cakes, oat bran, and barley. Fats and oils will increase the diarrhea that is a part of colitis. Spicy foods and coffee should also be avoided. Protein should be eaten as poultry, not red meat. Meats should be broiled or baked without the skin. Never fry your foods. Eat plenty of vegetables, preferably raw, but lightly steamed, if necessary.

Also drink the juice from cabbage, carrots, and other green drinks daily. All fruit or fruit juices should be eaten with meals, never on an empty stomach. Vegetable juices are preferable. A juicer is a small investment to make for your health's sake.

Crohn's disease is chronic inflammation of a section of the digestive tract. The inflammation goes through all the layers of the intestinal tissue and affects adjacent lymph nodes. As the inflammation heals, scar tissue forms and this can narrow the passageway for food.

Crohn's disease symptoms include (1) loss of energy, (2) weight loss, (3) anemia, (4) cramping, severe at times, (5) lower-right abdominal pain, (6) fever, (7) malassimilation which can weaken the immune system, (8) diarrhea, and (9) blood in the stool.

Crohn's disease typically hits around age twenty, and while the cause is unknown, it is thought that food allergies may be the trigger. If the disease is left untreated, many things can happen. Peritonitis may occur if the intestinal wall leaks, cancer could develop, and bowel function usually deteriorates.

Take fluids freely and eat nonacidic foods. Include cabbage, Brussels sprouts, carrots, spinach, kale, turnips, broccoli, and celery in your diet. Avoid all animal products, alcohol, coffee, chocolate, tobacco, pepper, spicy foods, fried and greasy foods, and carbonated drinks.

Again, learn to control your reaction to stress. It is easy to advise someone to avoid stress, but in today's society it is a fact of life. Although we cannot avoid stress, we can learn to react differently to it. Rest during an attack of Crohn's disease and use heat to lessen abdominal pain.

Diverticulitis is inflammation of the mucous membranes in the colon, forming small pouches or sacs in weakened areas of the alimentary tract. Constipation is what causes small pouches to form. The pouches cause trouble when they become filled with waste matter and then become inflamed or infected. Poor diet and stress increase the problem. If there is a history of diverticulitis in your family, your risk of developing the disease is increased. Obesity, coronary artery disease, and gallbladder problems also seem to be linked to the disorder.

Symptoms of diverticulitis are (1) diarrhea or constipation, (2) pain that is relieved after passing gas or a bowel movement, (3) cramps, and (4) nausea.

Enemas can help relieve the symptoms of this disorder. Fasting several days a month can also help cleanse the body of toxins and regulate the bowels.

HERBS HELPFUL FOR INTESTINAL COMPLAINTS

These herbs and the herbal remedies that follow are helpful for dealing with intestinal disorders: licorice root, peppermint, plantain, marshmallow root, slippery elm, bugleweed, wild yam, chickweed, and papaya.

LICORICE ROOT
Glycyrrhiza glabra

OTHER NAMES: Sweetwood, liquorice.
PART USED: Dried root.
SIGNATURE: The length of the root and the sweet taste are its signature.

Licorice is antiulcer, antispasmodic, antiseptic, antiinflammatory, antifungal, antibacterial, and antimicrobial. Here the herb is used to treat diverticulitis, gastritis, and colitis. It cleanses the colon and increases the mucous-secreting cells of the digestive system. This helps increase the life of intestinal cells and aids in the microcirculation of the gastrointestinal lining. Licorice root is also used to help relieve stress.

The coumarins in licorice act as a laxative; other components are glycyrrhizin, asparagine, and terpenes. The minerals present are magnesium, potassium, phosphorus, tin, and silicon. It also contains fat, protein, biotin, PABA, inositol, and choline, as well as vitamins B_1, B_2, B_3, B_5, B_6 C, D, and E with traces of A.

Caution: Do not use licorice root if you have high blood pressure or heart disease.

LICORICE TEA

Place 2 teaspoons of licorice root in a cup. Pour 1 cup of boiling water over the herb and steep 10 to 15 minutes. Strain and drink several cups per day.

LICORICE ROOT TINCTURE

Place 1 ounce of licorice root in a pint jar. Fill the container with vodka or brandy. Allow the mixture to steep in a sunny window for at least two weeks. Strain and place in a sterile container. Take 1 teaspoon of the tincture in 1 cup of hot water or juice, or add it to other herbal teas. Drink several cups per day, as desired.

LICORICE ROOT CAPSULES

1 tablespoon of powdered licorice root
1 tablespoon of powdered black cohosh
1 tablespoon of powdered ginseng

Mix the herbs and place thcm in #00 capsules. Take 6 capsules daily in divided doses.

LICORICE-GINSENG DIARRHEA TREATMENT

Licorice combined with ginseng helps rejuvenate the digestive system by increasing fluids and enzymes and reducing inflammation. Mix equal parts of ginseng and licorice root, and fill #00 capsules. Take 2 capsules three times daily with meals.

Make tea, if you wish, by placing 1 teaspoon each of the herbs in a cup and pouring 1 cup of boiling water over them. Cover and steep 15 minutes. Drink with every meal.

PEPPERMINT
Mentha piperita

OTHER NAMES: Brandy, lamb mint, American mint.
PART USED: Leaves and flowering top.
SIGNATURE: The herb grows in wet or damp soil.

Peppermint has long been used as a treatment for diarrhea, flatulence, and bloating. It is helpful because it releases the production of digestive fluids and shrinks inflamed tissue. It will help with loss of appetite and has the ability to loosen and eliminate hardened mucus.

Peppermint is considered to be a stimulant, astringent, and antispasmodic; it is also antimicrobial. It contains the minerals calcium, iron, magnesium, sodium, potassium, phosphorus, and tin, along with protein and vitamins A, B_3, and C. Its chemical components are methyl acetate, terpenes, menthone, menthol, tannic acid, and volatile oils.

Caution: Peppermint may interfere with iron absorption.

PEPPERMINT GINSENG TEA

2 tablespoons of ginseng
2 tablespoons of peppermint

Place 1 teaspoon of the herb mixture in a cup. Pour 1 cup of boiling water over the herbs and cover. Allow to steep 15 minutes. Strain and drink with every meal.

PEPPERMINT SYRUP

1 ounce of peppermint
2 ounces of goldenseal
$1/2$ pound of butternut bark

Use this as a treatment for sluggish bowels. Steep the herbs in 1 quart of boiling water for about an hour. Strain and add 2 pounds of sugar. Add 2 ounces of glycerin, shake well, and store in a sterile container. Take 1 teaspoon morning and night. Ten drops of *Cascara sagrada* tincture may be added to each dose of the syrup, if desired.

PEPPERMINT CAPSULES

2 tablespoons of powdered peppermint
2 tablespoons of powdered papaya (pawpaw)
2 tablespoons of powdered plantain

Place the mixed herbs in #00 capsules. Take 2 capsules three times daily.

PLANTAIN
Plantago major

OTHER NAMES: Ripplegrass, ribwort, wagbread, common plantain, white-man's-foot, cart-track plant, broadleaf plantain, cuckoo's bread, Englishman's foot.
PART USED: Seeds, leaves, and root.
SIGNATURE: Erect flowering spikes are plantain's signature.

Plantain can be used to treat Crohn's disease, ulcers, chronic colitis, gastritis, enteritis, diarrhea, dysentery, and inflammatory intestinal conditions. Plantain regulates colonic flora and absorbs toxins from the intestines. It is considered antidiarrheal and antiinflammatory, and it promotes friendly bacteria in the colon. The herb relieves inflammation of the intestinal tract as well as reducing the transit time of foods. That is, plantain adds bulk to the stool while soothing the lining of the digestive system.

It is considered an alterative, astringent, diuretic, and antiseptic. Plantain relieves the pain of intestinal ulcers and digestive complaints.

The minerals present in plantain are magnesium, manganese, calcium, cobalt, chromium, selenium, silicon, zinc, potassium, phosphorus, and sodium. It is very high in vitamin C.

PLANTAIN TINCTURE

The whole plant, including the root system, seeds, and leaves, is used to prepare the tincture. Fill a quart jar about half-full, pressing down on the herb. Finish filling the jar with vodka or brandy. Allow the mixture to steep in a sunny area for two to three weeks before straining. Store it in a sterile container. Take 1 teaspoon of the tincture in 1 cup of hot water several times daily.

HEMORRHOID TREATMENT

Prepare a tea of 4 to 6 fresh leaves of plantain to each cup of boiling water. Use 1 to 2 teaspoons of the dried herb if fresh leaves are not available. Steep until cool. Strain and store. Inject 1 tablespoon of the tea into the rectum after each bowel movement.

PLANTAIN COMBINATION CAPSULES

> 1 tablespoon of powdered plantain
> 1 tablespoon of powdered bugleweed
> 1 tablespoon of powdered marshmallow root

Mix the powdered herbs and fill #00 capsules. Take 2 capsules three times daily.

PLANTAIN TEA

Place 4 to 5 leaves of fresh plantain in a cup. Pour 1 cup of boiling water over the herb and cover. Steep 15 minutes. Drink with every meal. Sweeten with honey, if desired.

MARSHMALLOW ROOT
Althaea officinalis

OTHER NAMES: Althea root, sweetweed, white mallow, mortification root.
PART USED: Whole plant and root.
SIGNATURE: The herb's sweet taste and the fact that it grows in wet areas are its signature.

Marshmallow root relieves gastritis, gastric ulcers, and inflammation of the gastrointestinal system. Marshmallow acts as a demulcent and emollient, so it is very soothing for inflammations. It also lessens the transit time of foods through the intestinal tract. Marshmallow contains polysaccharides which coat the mucous membranes of the digestive tract. It also absorbs, binds, and eliminates toxins from the digestive system and regulates the intestinal flora.

Minerals present in marshmallow are calcium, chromium, selenium, magnesium, iron, phosphorus, potassium, sodium, and tin. The root also has protein and about 164 mg of vitamin C. The amount of sodium available in marshmallow is more than average for most medicinal herbs.

MARSHMALLOW TEA

1 tablespoon of marshmallow root
1 tablespoon of crushed fenugreek seeds

Mix the root and seeds. Add 1 teaspoon of the herb mixture to a cup, and pour 1 cup of boiling water over the herbs. Steep 10 to 15 minutes, covered. Strain and drink several cups per day, as desired.

MARSHMALLOW CAPSULES

1 tablespoon of powdered marshmallow root
1 tablespoon of powdered plantain
1 tablespoon of powdered slippery elm

Mix the powdered herbs and fill #00 capsules. Take 6 to 8 capsules during the day to soothe inflammations and ulcers and to eliminate toxins in the intestinal tract.

SLIPPERY ELM
Ulmus rubra (Ulmus fulva)

OTHER NAMES: Red elm, Indian elm, moose elm, American elm.
PART USED: Dried bark or fresh inner bark.
SIGNATURE: The mucilaginous substance (revealed when chewed) and the color of the bark are slippery elm's signature.

Slippery elm can be used to treat Crohn's disease and any inflammatory disease of the colon. It is considered an astringent, demulcent, and emollient. The astringent properties shrink inflamed tissue, decrease food's transit time in the alimentary tract, and regulate the intestinal flora. The herb absorbs toxins in the digestive system. It is good for diarrhea.

Slippery elm will stay down in a cancerous stomach when nothing else will, if used as a gruel. It soothes, heals, and cleanses the lining of the digestive tract.

The minerals present in slippery elm are magnesium, calcium, manganese, sodium, tin, potassium, phosphorus, iron, cobalt, zinc, selenium, and chromium. It also contains protein, and vitamins A, B_3, and K, and bioflavonoids.

COLD SLIPPERY ELM TEA

As a treatment for inflammation of the digestive tract, slippery elm is a valuable herb. The tea is best made cold. The liquid becomes too thick if hot water is used.

Place 1 ounce of slippery elm bark in 2 quarts of cold water. Allow the bark to steep several hours. Strain and refrigerate. Drink the cold tea freely throughout the day.

To soothe the lower intestine, use the tea as an enema.

SLIPPERY ELM CONSTIPATION TREATMENT

Prepare a tincture of fresh slippery elm bark to use as an aid for constipation. Place 1 ounce of fresh bark into a pint jar. Fill the container to the top with vodka or brandy. Place in a sunny area and allow to steep for two weeks. Strain and store in a sterile bottle. Take 1 tablespoon of the tincture in 8 ounces of water, three times daily until you obtain relief.

COMBINATION CAPSULES
FOR INTESTINAL COMPLAINTS

1 tablespoon of powdered slippery elm
1 tablespoon of powdered licorice root
1 tablespoon of powdered plantain
1 tablespoon of powdered lobelia
1 tablespoon of powdered comfrey root
1 tablespoon of powdered rhubarb root

Mix the powdered herbs and fill #00 capsules. Take 6 to 8 capsules per day.

BUGLEWEED
Lycopus virginicus

OTHER NAMES: Meadow bugle, Gypsy wort, water horehound.
PART USED: Top.
SIGNATURE: The herb grows in wet or moist areas.

Bugleweed is used as a treatment for colitis, diarrhea, dysentery, and intestinal gas. It contains hemostatic properties and helps relieve pain.

Considered an astringent, it can shrink tissues that are inflamed. It is also an expectorant, diuretic, alterative, nervine, antacid, and diaphoretic. Bugleweed contains marrubiin, resin, tannin, and volatile oils. Iron, potassium, fat, and vitamins A, B complex, C, and E are also present.

It can be used as a tincture, an infusion, a decoction, or in capsule form. The alterative and tonic properties are very soothing to the mucous membranes, which helps relieve intestinal inflammation.

BUGLEWEED TINCTURE

Place 1 ounce of the herb in a pint jar. Cover the herb completely with vodka or brandy. Place the jar in a warm area for about two weeks, shaking daily. Strain and store. Take up to 1 teaspoon in hot water or other herbal teas. Drink two times daily for a week.

BUGLEWEED CAPSULES

1 tablespoon of powdered bugleweed
1 tablespoon of powdered marshmallow
1 tablespoon of powdered slippery elm
1 tablespoon of powdered peppermint

Mix the powdered herbs and fill #00 capsules. Take 2 capsules three times daily.

WILD YAM
Dioscorea villosa

OTHER NAMES: China root, rheumatism root, colic root.
PART USED: Root.
SIGNATURE: The knotted and contorted root stalk and the fact that it has vines are its signature.

Wild yam can be used for any inflammatory condition. It relieves inflammation of the digestive tract. Wild yam contains properties similar to those of steroids, but the herb must be digested and processed by the body to become effective as a steroid.

It is considered antispasmodic and antiinflammatory and has a balancing effect on the whole digestive system. The herb is effectively used for spasms of the colon and for relieving pain.

Wild yam contains the steroidal glycosides sapogenin and yamogenin; its mucilaginous properties come from polysaccharides. The tannin found in the plant is considered to have astringent properties. The minerals present are magnesium, cobalt, calcium, sodium, tin, potassium, phosphorus, manganese, and iron.

WILD YAM TINCTURE

Place 1 ounce of wild yam in a pint jar. Cover the herb completely with vodka or brandy. Allow the jar to stand in a sunny window for two weeks. Strain and bottle. Add 1 to 2 teaspoons of the tincture to hot water or other herbal teas.

WILD YAM TEA

> 1 tablespoon of wild yam root
> 1 tablespoon of papaya leaves
> 1 tablespoon of peppermint

Place 1 to 2 teaspoons of the herb mixture in a cup. Pour 1 cup of boiling water over the herbs and allow the mixture to steep 15 minutes. Strain and drink several times daily with meals.

WILD YAM CAPSULES

> 1 tablespoon of powdered wild yam root
> 1 tablespoon of powdered slippery elm
> 1 tablespoon of powdered ginger

Mix the powdered herbs and fill #00 capsules. Take 2 capsules morning and evening.

CHICKWEED
Stellaria media

OTHER NAMES: Scarwort, satin flower, starweed, stitchwort, adder's mouth, star chickweed, starwort.

PART USED: Upper part.

Chickweed is used mainly to prevent constipation and to provide needed minerals and vitamins in tonic form. Chickweed increases digestive fluids and soothes inflamed tissue. It also gives bulk to the stool and reduces mucus buildup in the lungs and other organs while decreasing its thickness. It helps with elimination and detoxifies the gastrointestinal system. The herb is frequently used as a vitamin C supplement because of its high content of the vitamin.

Chickweed increases the absorption of minerals from the digestive tract and can be eaten as a potherb or added to salads, soups, stews, and casseroles. The vitamin C content is best obtained by adding it to salads.

The nutrients available in chickweed are copper, potassium, iron, cobalt, calcium, magnesium, selenium, sodium, zinc, phosphorus, manganese, silicon, choline, inositol, rutin, and potash salts. It also contains PABA, biotin, pantothenic acid, and vitamins A, B_1, B_2, B_3, B_6, B_{12}, C, and D.

CHICKWEED TINCTURE

Place a large handful of fresh chickweed in a pint jar. Cover completely with vodka or brandy. Let the jar stand in a warm sunny area for two weeks, shaking it daily. Strain and place in a sterile container. Add 1 tablespoon of the tincture to 1 cup of hot water or herbal tea; drink with meals.

CHICKWEED COMBINATION CAPSULES

> 1 tablespoon of powdered chickweed
> 1 tablespoon of powdered cascara sagrada
> 1 tablespoon of powdered alfalfa

Mix the powdered herbs and fill #00 capsules. Take 2 capsules twice daily for a week.

CHICKWEED TEA

Add several tablespoons of fresh chickweed or several teaspoons of dried chickweed to a cup. Pour 1 cup boiling water over the herb. Steep 10 to 15 minutes, covered. Strain and drink as often as desired.

DANDELION
Taraxacum officinale

OTHER NAMES: Cankerwort, lion's tooth, blowball, wild endive, common dandelion.
PART USED: Whole plant: leaves, flowers, and root.
SIGNATURE: The color of the flower is its signature.

Dandelion is widely used to relieve indigestion, constipation, and circulatory and glandular disorders. It increases bile and digestive fluids. The root is especially used for constipation. As a tonic, dandelion increases the body's efficiency in elimination while detoxifying the gastrointestinal system. The herb also works as a great blood purifier.

Dandelion regulates the intestinal flora, producing helpful bacteria that kill ingested toxins. The flavonoids present soothe the digestive tract. Its mineral content is well balanced with calcium, iron, zinc, sodium, sulfur, potassium, phosphorus, magnesium, manganese, silicon, and tin. Vitamins present are PABA, pantothenic acid, A, B complex, C, and E. It also contains protein. Add the herb to your daily diet by using the leaves in salads or as a potherb. The flower can be made into jelly or wine. The root may be used as a coffee substitute or may be added to chicory for a coffee blend.

DANDELION TEA

Place several teaspoons of dandelion root in a cup. Pour 1 cup of boiling water over the herb. Cover and steep a half-hour. Strain and drink three times daily until you obtain relief.

DANDELION TINCTURE

Place 1 ounce of dried dandelion root in a pint jar. Add vodka or brandy. Cover and let the jar stand in a warm area for two weeks. Strain and place in a sterile container. Add 1 tablespoon to hot water, and drink several times daily until relieved of constipation.

DANDELION TONIC CAPSULES

1 tablespoon of powdered dandelion root
1 tablespoon of powdered pau d'arco

1 tablespoon of powdered purslane
1 tablespoon of powdered slippery elm

Mix the powdered herbs and fill #00 capsules. Take 2 capsules three times daily for a month.

PAPAYA
Carica papaya

OTHER NAMES: Pawpaw, melon tree, custard apple.
PART USED: Fruit, juice, leaves, seeds, and sap.
SIGNATURE: The yellow milky juice and the color of the ripe fruit are its signature.

Papaya is rich in enzymes that break down protein in the body. It can be used for all stomach disorders and impaired digestion. As a digestive aid, it helps the body convert proteins into amino acids and peptides while also digesting carbohydrates and fats.

Do not overuse papaya or any other digestive enzyme. The papain in the herb contains compounds similar to those that compose the human body. Excess papain can cause holes in your digestive tract and inflame intestinal tissues.

The digestive enzymes in papaya include chymopapain, lipase, lysozyme, and papain. Volatile oils, pectin, polysaccharides, and resin are also present. Minerals include calcium, sodium, silicon, phosphorus, cobalt, magnesium, potassium, and selenium. Also present are vitamins A, B_1, B_2, B_3, C, and D.

PAPAYA TINCTURE

Use papaya leaves to prepare the tincture. Place 1 ounce of dried leaves in a pint jar. Fill the jar with vodka or brandy. Allow the mixture to stand in a sunny area for two weeks. Strain and store in a clean container. Take 1 teaspoon of the tincture in 1 cup of hot water, or add it to other herbal teas.

PAPAYA TEA

Add 1 teaspoon of dried papaya leaves to 1 cup of boiling water. Steep covered for 15 minutes. Strain and drink once a day for a week.

PAPAYA CAPSULES

1 tablespoon of powdered papaya leaves
1 tablespoon of powdered licorice root
1 tablespoon of powdered fenugreek
1 tablespoon of powdered ginger

Mix the powdered herbs and fill #00 capsules. Take 2 capsules twice a day for two weeks. Discontinue taking them for two weeks, and resume for several more weeks, as needed.

PAPAYA-PEPPERMINT TEA

1 tablespoon of dried peppermint leaves
1 tablespoon of dried papaya leaves
1 tablespoon of dried chickweed

Add 1 teaspoon of the herb mixture to a cup. Pour 1 cup of boiling water over the herb mixture. Allow to steep for 15 minutes. Strain and use honey as a sweetener, if desired. Drink 2 cups daily for one week.

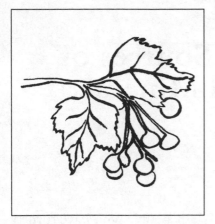

Cranberry

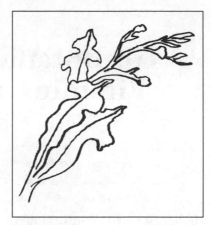

Milk Thistle

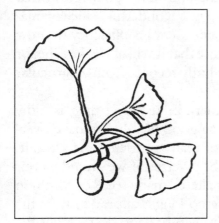

Ginkgo

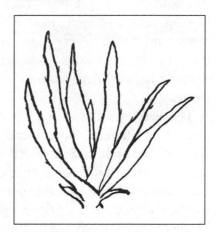

Aloe Vera

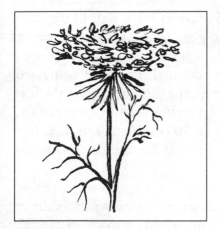

Queen Anne's Lace

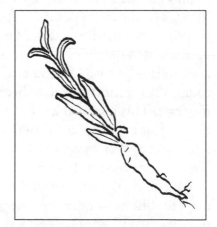

Horseradish

10. Botanical Sources of Vitamins and Minerals

Medicinal herbs require time to work. Many people who have turned to natural herbs as a health aid give them up after discovering that healing results come slowly. The body is a wonderful, efficient machine, and it takes a very long time for a nutrient insufficiency to show up as a serious disorder. So, it makes sense that it will also take time for a particular medicinal herb to help the body recover from a particular illness.

The Western diet, especially the American fast-food diet, is sadly lacking in vitamins and minerals vital to good health. We have overworked our soils and depleted them of many nutrients. As a result, many of us suffer illnesses that could be reversed if we attend to our food sources. Since we have genetically altered many seeds of common foods, we may have a price to pay. We no longer appear to have the biodiversity of plants we had just a few centuries ago. Remember the potato famine in Ireland? That was brought about in part because of the lack of variety in potato crops in 19th century Ireland. In this century, we have also limited our farms and gardens to a very few varieties of available vegetables and fruits. Although over 80,000 plant foods are available, only 3 percent of these potential foods are cultivated today. Plant extinctions have been running at a thousand times the former rate. This means that about 27,000 plants a year become extinct. Today, just twenty plant varieties make up 90 percent of our diet. Is it any wonder that maintaining good health has become an important interest for everyone?

We could take vitamin and mineral supplements, and we probably need to. But most nutrition supplements are produced synthetically in pharmaceutical laboratories. Since the human body is made of natural, organic material, it more readily metabolizes organic foods. Many of the chemical components used to manufacture these bottled nutrients as well as the additives and excipients that remain in the tablet or capsule cannot be usefully digested. In contrast, we easily eliminate any waste products of most natural plant foods we ingest through the alimentary system. What the body cannot and does not use, the body usually disposes of. But many synthetic additives and by-products linger in the body. The body does not know what to do with them. So, it stores them somewhere, often in the liver. The body simply does the best it can to protect us.

We would not pump water into the gas tank of a car. So, why would we ingest nonfoods, nonnutritive synthetics, in the body? We receive enough undigestible substances and toxins through pollution and other things in our environment. Every day we soap and shampoo, lather and lotion, breathe and eat more chemicals than the body can deal with.

However, we can make sure that the foods we grow and eat are organic, whether we grow them ourselves or purchase them from farmers who garden organically. Plants provide the human body with a natural way to ensure that we get sufficient fuel to keep healthy. And the phytochemicals in plants help protect us from disease. Avoid processed foods and those with additives and artificial ingredients.

In this chapter, the herbs and foods listed under specific nutrients, like vitamin A or selenium, can easily be added to your daily diet. You can take herbs as supplements, add them to foods, or drink them in teas or infusions. You can powder them to fill capsules or dilute them in teas. If you wish, you can also preserve herbs in a tincture with alcohol or in honey or glycerin as syrups. See the section "How to Prepare Herbs" in the Introduction of this book (pp. 10–12) for different ways to prepare herbs. Many herbs can be combined in a cup of tea. Simply add honey to sweeten if the herb(s) is bitter. See the appropriate chapter in this book of the disease(s) or ailment(s) that concerns you for some helpful recipes using recommended nutritive and medicinal herbs.

Please note that some herbs, though rich in given nutrients, may be counterindicated for certain ailments. For instance, you must not take licorice root if you have high blood pressure or heart disease. Some herbs, like goldenseal, should only be taken on a short-term basis. Other herbs, like ephedra, should only be used by people with acute asthma attacks and under a physician's supervision. The herb could be fatal to someone with heart disease or if it is ingested in a large amount. Still other herbs may cause an allergic reaction in some people.

Also, some foods may work the same way. Although they are a source of valuable minerals and vitamins, white potatoes and other nightshade vegetables, for instance, should be avoided by most arthritis sufferers. People with diabetes mellitus must avoid foods that make their blood sugar go haywire. (See the list of "Foods That Normalize Blood Sugar" in chapter 2, "Diabetes Mellitus.")

All the serious illnesses and ailments discussed in this book should be treated by a physician. Consult a physician about any dietary modification or any herbs you plan to use. It is also important to note any pharmacological interactions the herbs may have with any prescription drugs you may be taking. These herb and food remedies are not to be considered a substitute for a treatment regimen or medical care by a qualified physician. During pregnancy, it's best to avoid using medicinal herbs. Do not give herbs to young children.

Remember that many vitamins and minerals work best in combination, often synergistically. B-complex vitamins, for instance, require the presence of all the essential B vitamins to work effectively. Also, some nutrients, like iron and zinc, need to be taken at different times of day so that they do not knock out each other's effect. You may want to consult a standard book on nutrition to understand these interactions. Generally, the nutrients and other chemical components of plants—herbs, fruits, vegetables, legumes, and grains—work in harmony. This makes them more effective in your body. But in a commercial supplement, they may not.

Nutrient Sources

Many herbs and foods are valuable sources of nutrients vital to good health and the treatment of disease. They also contain phytochemicals with disease-prevention and healing properties. Review the chapter(s) about the disease(s) or ailment(s) that concerns you, paying special attention to the chapter's list of "Recommended Nutrients" and the chapter's discussion of "Helpful Herbs." Then, turn to the appropriate vitamin or mineral in this chapter (10) under "Nutrients" (pp. 166–186) to find herbs and foods to add to your daily treatment regimen.

Nutrients listed here include vitamins A, B complex, B_1 (thiamine), B_2 (riboflavin), B_3 (niacin), B_5 (pantothenic acid), B_6 (pyridoxine), B_{12} (cyanocobalamin), biotin, folic acid, C (ascorbic acid), D, E, and K;

bioflavonoids; and the minerals calcium, chlorine, chromium, copper, iodine, iron, magnesium, manganese, phosphorus, potassium, selenium, silicon, sodium, sulfur, and zinc. Also, some herbal sources of hormones are given.

Nutrients Recommended for Diseases or Ailments

Nutrients especially helpful for **arthritis** include vitamin C, chlorine, sodium, calcium, and potassium. Avoid nightshade vegetables (tomatoes, peppers, eggplant, white potatoes). Check for food and other allergies. Do not take iron supplements. See chapter 1.

For **diabetes mellitus,** consult the lists of herbs and foods high in vitamins A and E, chromium, calcium, and magnesium. Also take apple pectin. Chapter 2 lists foods that help normalize blood sugar (pp. 35–36) as well as types of food to avoid (p. 33).

If you have **asthma,** select herbs and foods high in vitamins B_6, C, and E and the minerals copper, magnesium, manganese, and iron. Review chapter 3. Also, heed any food or chemical allergies you may have.

If you have **chronic fatigue syndrome,** eat foods and ingest herbs high in vitamins B complex and C, as well as calcium, selenium, and zinc. Take kelp since it is a rich source of minerals and include garlic, a natural antibiotic, in your diet. See chapter 4.

For disorders of the **female reproductive system,** include B-complex vitamins and protein in your diet. Also, calcium, zinc, and vitamins A, B_6, C and E may be helpful. For disorders of the **male reproductive system,** include these recommended nutrients: vitamins A, B complex, especially B_6, C; and zinc. See chapters 5 and 6, respectively.

In the treatment of **cancer,** include beta-carotene, vitamins A, B complex, especially B_3, C, and E, and the minerals calcium, magnesium, selenium, and zinc. Avoid eating foods high in iron, and do not take an iron supplement. Add kelp and garlic to your daily diet. Consult chapter 7; especially lists of foods to eat and to avoid (pp. 111–112).

For **heart and circulatory disorders** and high blood pressure, include vitamins B complex, C, and E, as well as calcium, magnesium, selenium, and zinc in your daily diet. Also, include supplements of coenzyme Q10, lecithin, kelp, garlic, apple pectin, and primrose. Also see chapter 8 for healthful juices to include and for discussion of foods to avoid if you have cardiovascular disease. Do not ingest licorice or ephedra.

For **intestinal complaints,** be sure to eat foods and herbs rich in vitamins A, B complex, E, and K. Also, take kelp, alfalfa, acidophilus, proteolytic enzymes, multidigestive enzymes, aloe vera juice, and comfrey pepsin. Consult chapter 9 for other foods to include in your daily diet and foods to avoid.

NUTRIENTS

VITAMINS

VITAMIN A, a fat-soluble vitamin, aids in night vision, helps maintain soft mucous membranes, and is essential for growth. It aids in the growth and repair of body tissues and skin. Vitamin A helps counter the effects of stress and pollution. Herbs and foods high in vitamin A may be helpful in the treatment of diabetes mellitus, disorders of the female reproductive system and the male reproductive system, cancer, and intestinal complaints.

HERBS HIGH IN VITAMIN A

Gotu Kola	Blessed Thistle	Violet Leaves and Flowers
Peppermint	Red Raspberry Leaves	Lamb's-quarter
Yellow Dock	Nettle	Parsley
Bearberry (Uva Ursi)	Dandelion Root	Dandelion Greens
Brewer's Yeast	Garlic	Eyebright

FOODS HIGH IN VITAMIN A

Carrots	Alfalfa	Pumpkin	Kale
Cabbage	Broccoli	Peaches	Mustard Greens
Barley	Cayenne Pepper	Yellow Squash	Swiss Chard
Parsley	Spinach	Apricots	Asparagus
Horseradish	Papaya	Sweet Potatoes	Okra
Cantaloupe	Spirulina		

VITAMIN B COMPLEX helps maintain healthy skin, eyes, and hair; a healthy nervous system; and muscle tone in the gastrointestinal tract. Vitamin B complex is essential for the body's energy production by aiding in the conversion of carbohydrates to glucose. These vitamins are also necessary for the body's metabolism of protein and fats. All the B vitamins work in concert. So, a shortage of any one B vitamin can affect the function of the rest. B-complex vitamins help elevate mood and relieve depression and other nervous disorders. B-complex vitamins are water-soluble.

Vitamin B complex—B_1 (thiamine), B_2 (riboflavin), B_3 (niacin), B_5 (pantothenic acid), B_6 (pyridoxine), B_{12} (cyanocobalamin), biotin, and folic acid—may be helpful in the treatment of chronic fatigue syndrome, disorders of the female and male reproductive systems, cancer, heart and circulatory disorders, and intestinal complaints.

HERBS HIGH IN B-COMPLEX VITAMINS

Alfalfa: B complex
Black Cohosh: B_6
Blue Cohosh: B_3, B_5
Brewer's Yeast: B complex
Burdock: B_1, B_6, B_{12}, biotin
Catnip: B_1, B_2, B_3, B_5, B_6, B_{12}, biotin, folic acid
Cayenne Pepper (Capsicum): B_1, B_2, B_3, B_5, B_6, folic acid
Celery Seed: B complex
Chickweed: B_6, B_{12}, biotin
Dandelion: B_1, B_2, B_3, B_5, B_6, B_{12}, biotin, folic acid
Dong Quai Root: B_{12}
Eyebright: B_3, B_5, B_{12}
Fenugreek Seeds: B_1, B_2, B_3, B_5, B_6, B_{12}, biotin, folic acid
Garlic: B_1, B_2
Ginger: B_3, B_5, folic acid
Ginseng: B_1, B_{12}
Goldenseal: B complex
Hawthorn Berries: B_1, B_2, B_3, B_5, B_6, B_{12}, folic acid
Hops: B_6
Horehound: B complex
Horsetail: B_5
Kelp: B_1, B_2, B_3, B_5, folic acid
Licorice Root: B_1, B_2, B_3, B_5, B_6, biotin, folic acid
Mullein: B_2, B_5, B_{12}
Pumpkin Seeds: B_1, B_2, B_3

Red Clover Flowers: B_1, B_2, B_3, B_5, B_6, B_{12}, biotin, folic acid
Red Raspberry: B_1, B_3
Rose Hips: B_3
Thyme: B complex
White Oak Bark: B_{12}
Yerba Maté: B_5

VITAMIN B_1 (THIAMINE) maintains appetite and aids in carbohydrate metabolism. The vitamin enhances circulation and aids in blood formation. It is necessary for normal muscle tone of the stomach, intestines, and heart. Thiamine also helps steady the nerves.

Vitamin B_1 may be helpful in the treatment of heart and circulatory disorders and intestinal complaints. It is an important component of vitamin B complex.

HERBS HIGH IN VITAMIN B_1

Fenugreek	Brewer's Yeast	Kelp	Dandelion	Garlic

FOODS HIGH IN VITAMIN B_1

Brown Rice	Okra	Wheat Germ	Legumes
Salmon	Asparagus	Brussels Sprouts	Broccoli
Soybeans	Oatmeal	Plums	Peanuts
Peas	Nuts	Dried Prunes	Egg Yolks
Rice Bran	Raisins	Chickpeas	Sunflower Seeds
Organ Meats	Navy Beans	Kidney Beans	Fish

VITAMIN B_2 (RIBOFLAVIN) helps maintain normal growth in children. It is important in tissue respiration, red blood cell formation, and antibody production. The vitamin helps the body utilize carbohydrates, proteins, and fats. It helps maintain good vision and healthy skin, hair, and nails.

Vitamin B_2 may be helpful in the treatment of arthritis, diabetes mellitus, chronic fatigue syndrome, disorders of the female reproductive system, cancer, heart and circulatory disorders, and intestinal complaints.

HERBS HIGH IN VITAMIN B_2

Kelp	Fenugreek	Brewer's Yeast	Saffron	Garlic

FOODS HIGH IN VITAMIN B₂

Legumes	Spinach	Black Currants	Eggs
Cheese	Yogurt	Brussels Sprouts	Chicken
Milk	Asparagus	Nuts	Kidney Beans
Fish	Avocados	Poultry	Sunflower Seeds
Lean Beef	Swiss Cheese	Organ Meats	Peanuts

VITAMIN B₃ (NIACIN) helps lower cholesterol, improve circulation, and promote healthy skin. It aids in the metabolism of carbohydrates, proteins, and fats. It helps the functions of the nervous, digestive, and reproductive systems. The vitamin helps protect against recurrent nonfatal heart attacks.

Vitamin B₃ may be helpful in the treatment of arthritis, diabetes mellitus, chronic fatigue syndrome, disorders of the male reproductive system, heart and circulatory disorders, and intestinal complaints.

HERBS HIGH IN VITAMIN B₃

Hops	Burdock Seeds	Black Cohosh	White Willow
Feverfew	Chamomile	Peppermint	Mullein
Red Raspberry Leaves	Hydrangea	Parsley	Blueberry Leaves
Ginkgo Leaves	Red Clover	Gotu Kola	Fenugreek
Slippery Elm	Brewer's Yeast		

FOODS HIGH IN VITAMIN B₃

Asparagus	Carrots	Cheese	Watercress
Spirulina	Pork	Eggs	Wheat Germ
Cabbage	Beef	Tomatoes	Chicken
Barley	Broccoli	Cornmeal	Salmon
Alfalfa	Potatoes	Milk	Chicken Liver
Brown Rice	Peanuts	Beef Kidney	Whole Wheat
Sunflower Seeds	Tuna	Turkey	

VITAMIN B₅ (PANTOTHENIC ACID) aids in the function of the adrenal glands and helps maintain healthy skin and nerves. It aids in cell metabolism and in the maintenance of a healthy digestive tract.

Pantothenic acid may be helpful in the treatment of arthritis, asthma, chronic fatigue syndrome, disorders of the male reproductive system, and intestinal complaints.

HERBS HIGH IN VITAMIN B$_5$

Blue Cohosh	Kelp	Fenugreek Seeds	Brewer's Yeast
Catnip	Dandelion	Mullein	Horsetail
Cayenne Pepper	Eyebright	Ginger	
Hawthorn Berries	Red Clover Flowers		

FOODS HIGH IN VITAMIN B$_5$

Organ Meats	Egg Yolks	Whole Grains	Pork
Saltwater Fish	Legumes	Wheat Germ	Beans

VITAMIN B$_6$ (PYRIDOXINE) is involved in more bodily functions than any other nutrient. The vitamin aids in RNA and DNA synthesis. It helps the body produce antibodies, resist stress, and maintain emotional health. It enhances the immune system and increases energy. Vitamin B$_6$ helps maintain the balance of sodium and potassium in the body.

Vitamin B$_6$ may be helpful in the treatment of arthritis, diabetes mellitus, asthma, chronic fatigue syndrome, disorders of the reproductive system, heart and circulatory disorders, and intestinal complaints.

HERBS HIGH IN VITAMIN B$_6$

Burdock	Horehound	Hops	Goldenseal
Cayenne Pepper	Dandelion	Brewer's Yeast	Red Clover Flowers
Catnip	Fenugreek Seeds	Thyme	Alfalfa
Chickweed	Hawthorn Berries	Kelp	Celery Seeds

FOODS HIGH IN VITAMIN B$_6$

Tuna	Cantaloupe	Wheat Germ	Blackstrap Molasses
Carrots	Salmon	Avocados	Brown Rice

Chicken	Peas	Chickpeas	Whole Grains
Eggs	Spinach	Bananas	Cabbage
Shrimp	Sunflower Seeds	Navy Beans	Beans
Meat	Walnuts	Soybeans	Lentils

VITAMIN B$_{12}$ (CYANOCOBALAMIN) helps maintain a healthy nervous system and aids in the development of red blood cells. It helps maintain and regulate children's growth. It aids in the production of RNA and DNA. Vitamin B$_{12}$ is mostly found in animal protein and dairy products. It promotes healthy skin and high energy levels.

Vitamin B$_{12}$ may be helpful in the treatment of arthritis, asthma, diabetes mellitus, chronic fatigue syndrome, cancer, heart and circulatory disorders, and intestinal complaints.

HERBS HIGH IN VITAMIN B$_{12}$

Kelp	Brewer's Yeast	Dandelion	Mullein	Chickweed

FOODS HIGH IN VITAMIN B$_{12}$

Liver	Tofu	Salmon	Organ Meats
Mackerel	Beef Kidney	Herring	Cheese
Blue Cheese	Eggs	Clams	Pork
Swiss Cheese	Milk	Chicken	Seafood

BIOTIN, a coenzyme of the B-complex vitamins, aids in the production and oxidation of fatty acids, carbohydrates, and protein. It promotes healthy hair and skin.

Biotin may aid in the treatment of heart and circulatory disorders and intestinal complaints. Deficiencies are rare.

HERBS HIGH IN BIOTIN

Burdock	Chickweed	Fenugreek Seeds	Red Clover Flowers
Catnip	Dandelion	Brewer's Yeast	

FOODS HIGH IN BIOTIN

Egg Yolks	Liver	Brown Rice	Legumes
Whole Grains	Sardines	Poultry	Meat

FOLIC ACID (FOLACIN, FOLATE), a coenzyme of vitamin B complex, helps the body maintain healthy skin and a healthy digestive tract. It aids in the production of red and white blood cells and nucleic acid, which is essential for cell growth and reproduction. It helps maintain emotional health.

Folic acid may be helpful in the treatment of arthritis, asthma, chronic fatigue syndrome, disorders of the female reproductive system, heart and circulatory disorders, and intestinal complaints.

HERBS HIGH IN FOLIC ACID

Cayenne Pepper	Fenugreek Seeds	Hawthorn Berries	Red Clover Flowers
Catnip	Ginger	Kelp	Dandelion
Brewer's Yeast			

FOODS HIGH IN FOLIC ACID

Chicken Liver	Organ Meats	Whole Grains	Navy Beans
Chickpeas	Salmon	Milk	Oysters
Kidney Beans	Sunflower Seeds	Beef Liver	Green Leafy Vegetables

VITAMIN C (ASCORBIC ACID) must be supplied daily since the body does not store it. The vitamin is essential in maintaining healthy connective tissues and the integrity of cell walls. It aids in the formation of red blood cells. It promotes healing, acts as a natural antihistamine, helps reduce stress, and helps increase energy levels. Vitamin C may protect the body against flus and colds and some cancers. It helps maintain a healthy immune system. The vitamin also cools the body during exercise.

Vitamin C may be helpful in the treatment of arthritis, diabetes mellitus, asthma, chronic fatigue syndrome, cancer, disorders of the male reproductive system, heart and circulatory disorders, and intestinal complaints.

HERBS HIGH IN VITAMIN C

Aloe Vera Juice	Pine Needles	Parsley	Yellow Dock
Red Clover	Coltsfoot	Rose Hips	Bee Pollen

| Hops | Burdock Seeds | Red Raspberry Leaves | Alfalfa Seeds |

FOODS HIGH IN VITAMIN C

Broccoli	Horseradish	Lemons	Papaya
Cabbage	Paprika	Berries	Asparagus
Beet Greens	Currants	Kale	Lemons
Collard Greens	Mustard Greens	Onions	Red Peppers
Oranges	Grapefruit	Citrus Fruits	Strawberries
Peas	Swiss Chard	Tomatoes	Turnip Greens
Persimmons	Mangos	Cantaloupe	Green Peppers

VITAMIN D, a fat-soluble vitamin, can be absorbed by the skin from the sun's ultraviolet rays. It may also be ingested from food sources. Vitamin D helps strengthen bones and nourish muscles. It aids in the body's absorption of calcium from the intestines and helps the body break down and assimilate phosphorus. It is necessary for growth. The vitamin maintains a healthy nervous system and cardiovascular system.

Vitamin D may be helpful in the treatment of arthritis, diabetes mellitus, cancer, chronic fatigue syndrome, and intestinal complaints.

HERBS HIGH IN VITAMIN D

Alfalfa	Chickweed	Eyebright	Mullein
Red Raspberry	Rose Hips	Sarsaparilla	Thyme
Suma			

FOODS HIGH IN VITAMIN D

Herring	Mackerel	Salmon	Vitamin D–Fortified Dairy Products
Tuna	Egg Yolks	Organ Meats	Sardines
Watercress	Wheat Germ		

VITAMIN E (TOCOPHEROL), a fat-soluble vitamin, acts as an antioxidant that is necessary for cardiovascular health. It helps improve circulation, repairs tissue, and reduces the scars of wounded skin. It helps protect the body against environmental pollutants and toxins. It is essential for cell respiration. It helps maintain healthy eyes, lungs, heart, and muscles. It aids in reducing muscle cramps.

Vitamin E may be helpful in the treatment of arthritis, diabetes mellitus, asthma, chronic fatigue syndrome, disorders of the female reproductive system, heart and circulatory disorders, cancer, and intestinal complaints.

HERBS HIGH IN VITAMIN E

Kelp	Rose Hips	Rose Hips	Echinacea
Alfalfa	Dandelion Leaves	Skullcap	Goldenseal
Eyebright	Blue Cohosh	Linseeds	Ginseng
Horehound	Red Raspberry	Burdock Root	Suma

FOODS HIGH IN VITAMIN E

Sunflower Seeds	Whole Grains	Legumes	Eggs
Almonds	Green Leafy Vegetables	Sweet Potatoes	Cold-Pressed Vegetable Oils
Pecans	Wheat Germ	Watercress	Organ Meats
Dried Beans	Peanuts	Cornmeal	Sesame Seeds
Oatmeal	Brown Rice	Hazelnuts	Walnuts

VITAMIN K is necessary for blood clotting. It is vital for normal liver function; it converts glucose into glycogen for storage in the liver.

Vitamin K may be helpful in the treatment of cancer and intestinal complaints.

HERBS HIGH IN VITAMIN K

Shepherd's Purse	Chestnut Leaves	Alfalfa	Slippery Elm
Cornsilk	Gotu Kola		

FOODS HIGH IN VITAMIN K

Cabbage	Rye	Soybeans	Wheat
Broccoli	Oats	Brussels Sprouts	Cauliflower
Liver	Kale	Blackstrap Molasses	Spinach
Egg Yolks	Safflower Oil		

BIOFLAVONOIDS (VITAMIN P) are water-soluble and often appear with vitamin C in fruits and vegetables. Components of bioflavonoids include hesperidin, citrin, rutin, flavones, flavonals, quercetin, eriodictyol, and quercetrin. They promote circulation and preserve the capillary blood vessels. Bioflavonoids help lower cholesterol and stimulate bile production. They also act, with vitamin C, as an antioxidant and keep collagen healthy. They also have an antibacterial effect. Since the body cannot produce bioflavonoids, they must be included in the diet.

Bioflavonoids may be helpful in the treatment of arthritis, asthma, disorders of the female reproductive system, heart and circulatory disorders, and intestinal complaints.

HERBS HIGH IN BIOFLAVONOIDS

German Rue	Rose Hips	Hawthorn	Buckwheat Leaves

FOODS HIGH IN BIOFLAVONOIDS

Citrus Fruit Pulp	Peppers	Buckwheat	Black Currants
Apricots	Cherries	Grapefruit	Grapes
Lemons	Oranges	Prunes	Plums

MINERALS

CALCIUM helps maintain a regular heartbeat and provides the body with energy. It helps maintain strong teeth and bones and relieves muscle cramps. It is essential for healthy heart function and healthy blood. It assists in blood clotting and helps maintain a proper acid-alkali balance in the blood. It is important to muscle contraction and growth and nerve transmission. It helps reduce insomnia. A deficiency of calcium may cause heart palpitations, dermatitis, hypertension, nervousness, tooth decay, bone and joint disorders, numbness in arms and legs, muscle cramps, and increased cholesterol levels in the blood. Adequate magnesium and vitamin D are necessary for calcium absorption. The body requires calcium in a 2-to-1 ratio with phosphorus.

Calcium may be helpful in the treatment of arthritis, asthma, diabetes mellitus, chronic fatigue syndrome, heart and circulatory disorders, and intestinal complaints.

HERBS HIGH IN CALCIUM

Juniper Berries	Yellow Dock	Horehound	Black Cohosh
Gotu Kola	Marshmallow	Elecampane	White Oak Bark

Parsley	Eyebright	Fenugreek	Alfalfa
Ginseng	Chamomile	Thyme	Chickweed
Kelp	Rose Petals	Sage	Blue Cohosh
Dandelion	Hawthorn Berries	Angelica	Red Clover
Mullein	Anise Seeds	Buchu Leaves	Garlic

FOODS HIGH IN CALCIUM

Milk	Onions	Soybeans	Sardines
Egg Yolks	Dates	Salmon	Asparagus
Cayenne Pepper	Vegetable Tops	Green Leafy Vegetables	Red Raspberries
Apricots	Cheese	Almonds	Watercress
Cabbage	Figs	Molasses	Broccoli
Parsnips	Prunes	Buttermilk	Yogurt
Lettuce	Cranberries	Collards	Shellfish

CHLORINE (CHLORIDE) is an essential mineral that usually occurs in the body in a compound like sodium chloride or potassium chloride. Chlorine helps regulate the body's acid-alkali balance. It aids in the production of gastric juices in the stomach and helps in the digestion of proteins and fibrous foods. It stimulates the liver and helps rid the body of toxic wastes. It keeps joints and tendons healthy and helps distribute hormones. A deficiency may cause tooth or hair loss and impair digestion and muscle contraction.

Chlorine may be helpful in the treatment of arthritis and intestinal disorders.

HERBS HIGH IN CHLORINE

Kelp   Dulse   Sea Greens   Fennel

FOODS HIGH IN CHLORINE

Rye Flour   Ripe Olives   Table Salt   Seafood   Meats

CHROMIUM is involved in glucose metabolism and is needed for energy. It has been called glucose tolerance factor (GTF). It helps maintain stable blood sugar by aiding proper insulin utilization for people with diabetes as well as those with hypoglycemia. The mineral aids in synthesis of cholesterol, proteins, and fats. Chromium is necessary for a healthy heart.

Chromium may be helpful in the treatment of diabetes mellitus and heart and circulatory disorders.

HERBS HIGH IN CHROMIUM

Oatstraw	Catnip	Juniper Berries	Stevia Leaves
Red Clover Flowers	Hibiscus Flowers	Nettle	Brewer's Yeast
Ginkgo Leaves	Damiana Leaves	Spirulina	Lemongrass

FOODS HIGH IN CHROMIUM

Raisins	Cheese	Corn Oils	Mushrooms
Barley	Whole Grains	Dried Beans	Bee Pollen
Horseradish	Corn	Potatoes	Grapes

COPPER, a trace mineral found in all body tissues, aids in the formation of red blood cells and hemoglobin. It also helps form bones and forms elastin with zinc and vitamin C. It aids in healing, energy production, taste sensitivity, and in coloring hair and skin. The mineral is essential for the formation of collagen and RNA. It is important in protein metabolism and for healthy nerves.

Copper may be helpful in the treatment of arthritis and asthma.

HERBS HIGH IN COPPER

Dandelion	Violet	Thyme	Sarsaparilla
Mullein	Valerian	Marshmallow	Yarrow
Nettle	Elecampane	Juniper Berries	Red Clover
Saw Palmetto	Fenugreek	Horsetail	Ginseng
White Oak Bark	Sage	Burdock	Saint-John's-Wort

FOODS HIGH IN COPPER

Seafood	Whole Grains	Garlic	Organ Meats
Molasses	Artichokes	Beef Liver	Broccoli
Peanuts	Walnuts	Mushrooms	Lentils

Peas	Almonds	Soybeans	Cashews
Barley	Oatmeal	Salmon	Pecans
Legumes	Beets	Oranges	Wheat Germ

IODINE (IODIDE) is a trace mineral that aids in the development and functioning of the thyroid gland. It is an integral part of thyroxine, a hormone produced by the thyroid gland. It helps regulate energy, promotes growth, and stimulates the body's metabolism. It aids in mental function, speech, and healthy hair, skin, teeth, and nails. It helps the body synthesize and use cholesterol. Goiters indicate a serious iodine deficiency.

Iodine may be helpful in the treatment of arthritis, chronic fatigue syndrome, heart and circulatory disorders, and cancer.

HERBS HIGH IN IODINE

Kelp	Irish Moss	Iceland Moss	Garlic

FOODS HIGH IN IODINE

Mushrooms	Summer Squash	Sea Salt	Soybeans
Seafoods	Swiss Chard	Iodized Salt	Spinach
Sesame Seeds	Turnip Greens	Lima Beans	

IRON, a mineral present in every living cell, helps produce hemoglobin and oxygenate red blood cells. All iron in the body is combined with protein. Iron increases physical stamina, aids muscle function, and protects against anemia. Its enzymes promote protein metabolism. It aids in tissue respiration and requires calcium and copper to function. The mineral is important for growth and resistance to disease. It promotes a healthy immune system and proper digestive functions. Vitamin C aids in iron absorption.

Iron may be helpful in the treatment of arthritis, diabetes mellitus, chronic fatigue syndrome, disorders of the female reproductive system, and intestinal complaints.

HERBS HIGH IN IRON

Ginseng	Dandelion Root	Yellow Dock	Marigold
Kelp	Garlic	Chickory	Fenugreek

Parsley	Nettle	Horehound	Marshmallow
Borage	Slippery Elm	Violet	Thyme
Saint-John's-Wort	Hawthorn Berries	White Oak Bark	Juniper Berries
Valerian	Goldenseal	Mullein	

FOODS HIGH IN IRON

Blackberries	Oysters	Rye Flour	Kidney Beans
Potato Peelings	Liver	Bananas	Lima Beans
Whole Wheat	Walnuts	Dried Fruits	Pears
Black Cherries	Bean Sprouts	Soybeans	Pumpkin
Organ Meats	Fish	Poultry	Molasses
Egg Yolks	Avocados	Raspberries	Green Leafy Vegetables

MAGNESIUM, an essential mineral, is involved in many metabolic processes in the body. It counters the stimulative effect of calcium, playing an important role in muscle contractions and the transmission of nerve impulses. It helps in the body's absorption of calcium, phosphorus, potassium, and sodium and in the body's regulation of acid-alkaline balance. The mineral aids in bone growth and is necessary for the development of strong, hard, healthy teeth and bones. Magnesium helps the body adapt to cold and combat stress. It helps convert blood sugar into energy.

Magnesium may be helpful in the treatment of arthritis, asthma, diabetes mellitus, chronic fatigue syndrome, heart and circulatory disorders, and intestinal complaints.

HERBS HIGH IN MAGNESIUM

Kelp	Marigold	Ginseng	Orange Blossoms
Meadowsweet	Mullein	Parsley	Hawthorn Berries
Nettle	Saw Palmetto	Gotu Kola	Slippery Elm
Anise Seeds	Alfalfa	Juniper Berries	White Oak Bark
Horehound	Fenugreek	Red Clover	Cayenne Pepper
Toadflax	Borage	Saint-John's-Wort	Brewer's Yeast
Black Willow	Peppermint	Valerian	Garlic

FOODS HIGH IN MAGNESIUM

Dairy Products	Flaxseeds	Nuts	Raspberries
Blackstrap Molasses	Figs	Green Leafy Vegetables	Papaya
Meats	Grapefruit	Whole Grains	Goat's Milk
Seafood	Bananas	Millet	Egg Yolks
Apricots	Yellow Corn	Peaches	Kidney Beans
Avocado	Oranges	Black-Eyed Peas	Sesame Seeds
Apples	Lima Beans	Salmon	Brown Rice
Carrot Tops	Tofu	Coconut	Bean Sprouts

MANGANESE is needed by the nervous system. It aids in protein and fat metabolism and helps the body utilize vitamins B_1 and E. It works with B-complex vitamins to provide a feeling of well-being. It is necessary for normal skeletal development and for the formation of blood. It helps form mother's milk as well as urea, a part of urine. The mineral helps regulate blood sugar and maintain a healthy immune system.

Manganese may be helpful for arthritis, diabetes mellitus, asthma, chronic fatigue syndrome, and heart and circulatory disorders.

HERBS HIGH IN MANGANESE

Nasturtium Leaves	Bearberry (Uva Ursi)	Orange Blossoms	Chickweed
Mints	Juniper Berries	Chamomile	Rose Hips
Parsley	Yarrow	Eyebright	Catnip
Wintergreen	Saint-John's-Wort	Marshmallow	Hops
Gotu Kola	Valerian	Horehound	Irish Moss
Borage	Red Clover	Passionflower	Wood Betony
Ginseng	Garlic	Sage	Yellow Dock
Kelp	Hawthorn Berries	Alfalfa	Dandelion
Cayenne Pepper	Burdock	Fennel Seeds	

FOODS HIGH IN MANGANESE

Almonds	Watercress	Whole Grains	Spinach
Walnuts	Bee Pollen	Blueberries	Green Leafy Vegetables
Endive	Avocado	Raspberries	Seaweed

| Egg Yolks | Nuts | Legumes | Pineapple |
| Sprouts | Seeds | Dried Peas | |

PHOSPHORUS aids in heart contractions and kidney functions. The second most abundant mineral in the body, it is necessary for cell growth, formation of teeth and bones, and the transmission of nerve impulses. It should exist in a 2.5-to-1 calcium-to-phosphorus ratio. Phosphorus aids in the body's utilization of carbohydrates, proteins, and fats and in the production of energy. Both excess and insufficient amounts of phosphorus, calcium, and magnesium will have an adverse effect on the body. These three minerals need to be balanced for good health. Phosphorus deficiency is rare. This mineral is in most foods and carbonated beverages.

Phosphorus may be helpful in the treatment of arthritis, cancer, heart and circulatory disorders, and intestinal complaints.

HERBS HIGH IN PHOSPHORUS

Blue Cohosh	Siberian Ginseng	Marigold Flowers	Meadowsweet Flowers
Buchu Leaves	Brewer's Yeast	Calamus	Yerba Santa
Ginkgo Leaves	Sorrel	Peppermint	Garlic
Fennel Seeds	Chickweed	Yellow Dock	Milk Thistle Seeds
Caraway Seeds			

FOODS HIGH IN PHOSPHORUS

Cabbage	Salmon	Bran	Cauliflower
Corn	Okra	Soybeans	Barley
Pumpkin Seeds	Asparagus	Cranberries	Brussels Sprouts
Whole Grains	Dried Fruits	Horseradish	Watercress
Eggs	Poultry	Broccoli	Sesame Seeds

POTASSIUM helps maintain a healthy nervous system and a regular heart rhythm. It nourishes the muscular system and works with phosphorus to send oxygen to the brain. With sodium it helps regulate the body's water balance. It is necessary for normal growth, muscle contraction, and proper alkalinity of body fluids. It helps maintain steady blood pressure and regulates the transfer of nutrients to the cells. Potassium is in all vegetables and legumes.

Potassium may be helpful in the treatment of arthritis, diabetes mellitus, asthma, chronic fatigue syndrome, cancer, heart and circulatory disorders, and intestinal complaints.

HERBS HIGH IN POTASSIUM

Horseradish	Red Clover	Skullcap	Brewer's Yeast
Parsley	Sage	Bee Pollen	Yarrow
Dandelion Greens	Kelp	Blessed Thistle	Horsetail
Black Walnut Leaves	Summer Savory	Borage	American Centaury
Primrose Flowers	Hops	Alum Root	Birch Bark
Coltsfoot	Lemongrass	Nettle	Eyebright
Fennel Seeds	Dulse	Catnip	Carrot Tops
German Chamomile	Peppermint	Oak Bark	Queen Anne's Lace
Mullein	Feverfew	Plantain	Garlic

FOODS HIGH IN POTASSIUM

Blackberries	Blueberries	Almonds	Nuts
Bananas	Beet Greens	Cherries	Winter Squash
Broccoli	Corn	Cucumbers	Yams
Lima Beans	Black Currants	Carrots	Wheat Bran
Pecans	Peanuts	Brussels Sprouts	Apricots
Barley	Artichokes	Cauliflower	Grapefruit
Mushrooms	Mustard Greens	Onions	Sardines
Radishes	Prunes	Potatoes	Flounder
Peaches	Olives	Lemons	Tomatoes
Kale	Eggplant	Raisins	Salmon
Spinach	Honey	Figs	Orange Juice
Celery	Cabbage	Watercress	Blackstrap Molasses
Asparagus	Horseradish	Dairy Foods	Brown Rice
Legumes	Whole Grains	Avocado	Dates

SELENIUM, a natural antioxidant, helps maintain the elasticity of body tissue. It works with vitamin E to promote normal growth and health of the reproductive system. It aids in the function of the pancreas and helps maintain a healthy heart. It helps regulate blood pressure and prevents platelet aggregation. The mineral produces anti-bodies with vitamin E and helps protect the immune system. High concentrations of selenium are found in the pancreas, liver, and pituitary gland. Selenium prevents the conversion of free radicals into carcinogens by oxidation.

Selenium may be helpful in the treatment of arthritis, cancer, disorders of the reproductive system, heart and circulatory disorders, and intestinal complaints.

HERBS HIGH IN SELENIUM

Hibiscus Flowers	Buchu Leaves	Blessed Thistle	Black Cohosh
Yerba Santa	Yarrow Flowers	Althea Root	Sarsaparilla Root
Dog Grass	Valerian Root	Dulse	Brewer's Yeast
Milk Thistle	Barberry Root		

FOODS HIGH IN SELENIUM

Whole Grains	Chicken Liver	Dairy Products	Onions
Herring	Kidneys	Broccoli	Salmon
Pumpkin Seeds	Shellfish	Chicken	Tuna
Wheat Germ	Brown Rice	Brazil Nuts	Molasses
Sunflower Seeds	Sesame Seeds	Wheat Germ	

SILICON (SILICA) is necessary for the formation of healthy bones, collagen, and connective tissue. It helps maintain flexible arteries and prevent cardiovascular disease. The mineral helps maintain healthy skin, hair, and nails. Silicon counteracts the effects of aluminum in the body and may aid in the prevention of Alzheimer's disease. Horsetail grass, rich in silicon, is the only plant that has grown on earth for 280 million years.

Silicon may be helpful in the treatment of arthritis and heart and circulatory disorders.

HERBS HIGH IN SILICON

Horsetail Grass	Cornsilk	Chickweed	Gotu Kola
Dulse	Echinacea	Burdock Root	Thyme
Eyebright	Blue Cohosh	Lemongrass	Valerian
Ginger Root	Oatstraw	Goldenseal	Alfalfa

FOODS HIGH IN SILICON

Hard Drinking Water	Beets	Bell Peppers	Whole Grains
Green Leafy Vegetables	Soybeans	Seafood	Brown Rice

SODIUM is found in extracellular fluids, vascular fluids, and intestinal fluids. With potassium it helps maintain the body's acid-alkaline balance and water balance. It is necessary for muscle, nerve, and stomach functions. It counteracts acidosis and inhibits fermentation in the intestines. It helps keep other blood minerals soluble so that they will not become deposits in the bloodstream or joints. Sodium aids digestion, helps rid the body of carbon dioxide, and helps produce hydrochloric acid in the stomach. With chlorine it helps improve the health of the blood and lymphatic fluids. Sodium and potassium aid muscle contraction and transmission of nerve impulses.

Sodium may be helpful in the treatment of arthritis, chronic fatigue syndrome, and intestinal complaints.

HERBS HIGH IN SODIUM

Rose Hips	Irish Moss	Shepherd's Purse	Sassafras
Oatstraw	Peppermint	Dandelion Root	Sorrel
Buchu Leaves	Pennyroyal	Black Cohosh	Cleavers
Chamomile	Gotu Kola	Stinging Nettle	Coltsfoot
Wild Yam	Parsley	Black Willow	Bee Pollen
Kelp	Fennel Seeds	Slippery Elm	Alfalfa
Dulse	Meadowsweet	White Oak Bark	

FOODS HIGH IN SODIUM

Okra	Broccoli	Raspberries	Pomegranate
Grapefruit	Carrots	Brown Rice	Chinese Cabbage
Celery	Watercress	Strawberries	Leeks
Cabbage	Pumpkin	Pineapple	Pears
Cauliflower	Papaya	Watermelon	Squash
Milk Products	Whey	Seafood	Baking Powder

SULFUR is a mineral present in all plants and animals. It aids in tissue respiration, stimulates bile from the liver, and protects the body from toxins and radiation. It is essential for collagen synthesis and maintenance of healthy elastin in the skin. The mineral aids in metabolism and the health of the nervous system. It helps disinfect blood and protects the cell protoplasm.

Sulfur may be helpful in the treatment of cancer, chronic fatigue syndrome, and intestinal complaints.

HERBS HIGH IN SULFUR

Irish Moss	Silverweed	Nettle	Meadowsweet
Fennel Seeds	Coltsfoot	Pimpernel	Calamus
Garlic	Plantain Leaves	Eyebright	Horsetail
Shepherd's Purse	Cayenne Pepper		

FOODS HIGH IN SULFUR

Brussels Sprouts	Onions	Wheat Germ	Kale
Cabbage	Turnips	Eggs	Dried Beans
Watercress	Fish	Meat	Horseradish

ZINC occurs in larger amounts in the body than any other trace mineral except iron. It aids in healing, boosts the immune system, and protects the body against pollution. It may be helpful in preventing some cancers. It is required for protein synthesis and collagen formation. Zinc ensures the health of the male and female reproductive systems. It helps heal skin and wounds. It aids in taste sensitivity and helps protect the liver from damage by toxins.

Zinc may be helpful in the treatment of diabetes mellitus, chronic fatigue syndrome, cancer, disorders of the male and female reproductive systems, and heart and circulatory disorders.

HERBS HIGH IN ZINC

Bilberry	Kelp	Echinacea	Dulse
Brewer's Yeast	Pennyroyal	Nettle	Elecampane
Skullcap	Wild Yam	Irish Moss	Siberian Ginseng
Sage	Chickweed		

FOODS HIGH IN ZINC

Oysters	Organ Meats	Turkey	Seafood
Pumpkin Seeds	Whole Grains	Egg Yolks	Lamb Chops
Spirulina	Lima Beans	Liver	Mushrooms

Wheat Germ	Pecans	Sardines	Soybeans
Sunflower Seeds	Legumes	Soy Lecithin	

NATURAL HORMONES that may be helpful to the body are available from some botanical sources. These hormones may be helpful in the treatment of the female reproductive system. Consult the appropriate chapter for use.

HERBS HIGH IN FEMALE HORMONES

Star Grass	Linden Flowers	Sarsaparilla	Damiana
False Unicorn Root	Alfalfa	Pleurisy Root	Siberian Ginseng
Pussy Willow	Clover	Wild Yam Root	Garlic
Nettle			

FOODS HIGH IN FEMALE HORMONES

Sweet Potatoes	Carrots	Wheat Germ	Pomegranate Seeds

METRIC EQUIVALENTS

20 drops = $\frac{1}{5}$ teaspoon = 1 milliliter

100 drops = 1 dropper = 1 teaspoon = 5 milliliters

3 teaspoons = 1 tablespoon = 15 milliliters

1 cup = 0.24 liter = 8 fluid ounces = 1 (8-ounce) glass

1 pint = 2 cups = 0.48 liter

1 quart = 2 pints = 0.96 liter

1 gallon = 4 quarts = 3.84 liters

1 liter = 2.1 pints = 1.06 quarts

Index

189